Leukemia

A Comprehensive Guide to Understanding, Diagnosis, and Treatment

Ethan D. Anderson

Xspurts.com

A New Zealand Designed Product

Other Versions Available

Why limit yourself to just one format?

This book is now available in physical, digital, and audiobook options.

Choose the way you love to read and dive into the story today. You won't regret it!

Digital ISBN: 9781776969579
Physical ISBN: 9781776969562
Audio ISBN:

To obtain a different format of this book at a discounted price, please get in touch with us at:

http://isbn.xspurts.com/

Contents

Have Questions / Comments?

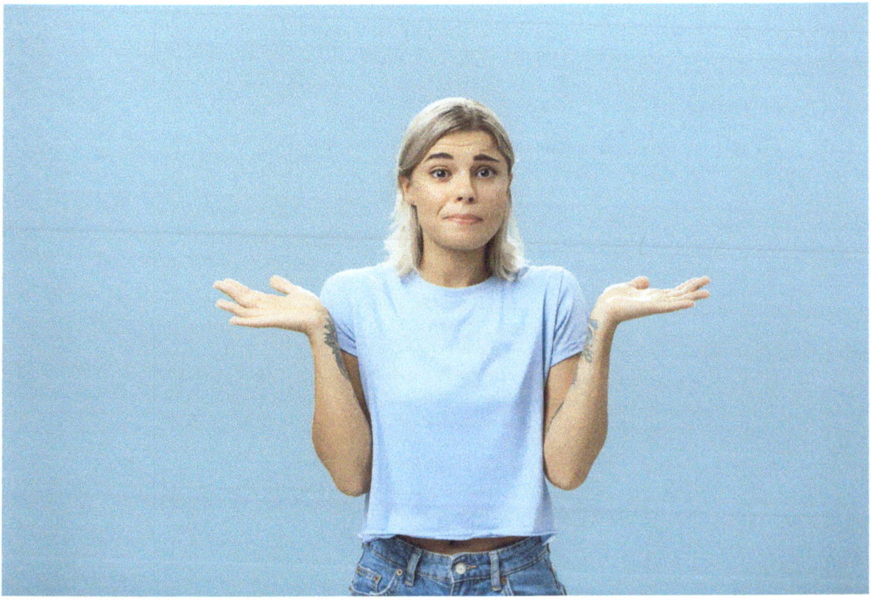

This book was designed to cover as much information as possible, but I know I have probably missed something, or some new amazing discovery has just come out.

If you notice something missing or have a question that I failed to answer, please get in touch and let me know. If I can, I will email you an answer and also update the book so others can also benefit from it.

Thanks For Being Awesome :)

Submit Your Questions / Comments At:

https://questions.xspurts.com

Get Free Stuff

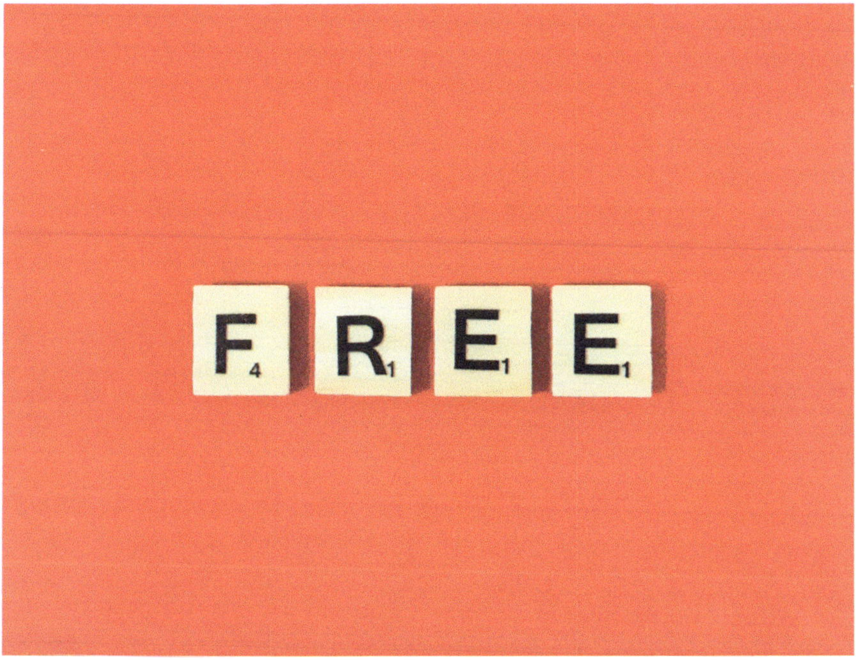

We love writing and have produced a huge number of books.

For being one of our amazing readers, we would love to offer you more books we have created, 100% free.

To claim this limited time special offer, simply go to the site below and enter your name and email address.

You will then receive loads (as we love our readers so much :) of our great books, content and audio direct to your email account, 100% free!

Get Loads of FREE Stuff at:

https://free.xspurts.com

Chapter One

Introduction

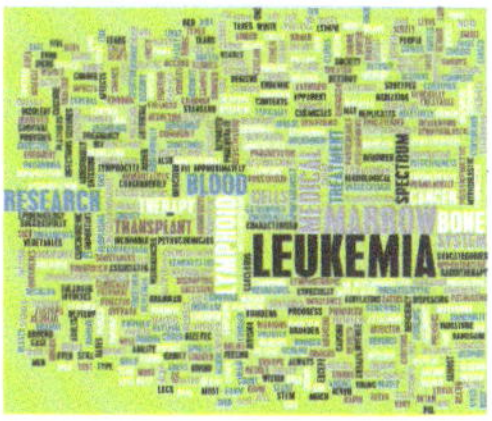

Leukemia is a complex and serious disease that affects millions of people around the world. It is a type of cancer that affects the blood and bone marrow, and it can be life-threatening if left untreated. Despite its severity, many people still have misconceptions and misunderstandings about Leukemia, which can cause fear and anxiety.

This book is designed to provide you with everything you need to know about Leukemia. Whether you or a loved one has been diagnosed with the disease, or you just want to learn more about it, this book is a comprehensive guide that covers all aspects of Leukemia.

We will explore the various types of Leukemia, the causes and risk factors, the symptoms and diagnosis, the different treatment options available, and the latest research and advancements in the field.

With this book, you will gain a deeper understanding of Leukemia and be equipped with the knowledge and resources to make informed decisions about your health.

What is

Leukemia

?

Leukemia is a type of cancer that affects the blood and bone marrow, the spongy tissue inside bones where blood cells are produced. Leukemia can affect both children and adults, and there are several different types of Leukemia that are classified based on the specific type of blood cell that is affected and how quickly the disease progresses.

Leukemia is a result of abnormal cell growth in the bone marrow, which can lead to an overproduction of immature or abnormal white blood cells that are unable to function properly. These cells can accumulate in the blood and other tissues, interfering with the normal functioning of organs and systems in the body.

The symptoms of Leukemia can vary depending on the type and stage of the disease, but may include fatigue, weakness, fever, frequent infections, easy bruising or bleeding, swollen lymph nodes, and weight loss. It is important to seek medical attention if these symptoms persist or if you experience any other unusual symptoms.

Treatment options for Leukemia may include chemotherapy, radiation therapy, targeted therapy, and stem cell transplantation. The choice of treatment will depend on the specific type of Leukemia, the stage of the disease, and other factors such as age and overall health.

While Leukemia can be a serious and life-threatening disease, advances in treatment have led to improved outcomes and increased survival rates for many patients. It is important to stay informed about Leukemia and to work closely with your healthcare team to manage the disease and optimize your chances for successful treatment and recovery.

Definition and Types

Leukemia is a type of cancer that affects the blood-forming cells in the bone marrow. It is characterized by the abnormal production of immature or damaged white blood cells that do not function properly. This disease can be divided into several types based on the rate of progression and the type of white blood cells that are affected.

Acute lymphoblastic leukemia (ALL) is the most common type of leukemia in children. It is a fast-growing cancer that affects the lymphoid cells in the bone marrow and blood. The symptoms of ALL may include fatigue, fever, bone pain, joint pain, and enlarged lymph nodes. Treatment for ALL typically involves chemotherapy, radiation therapy, and stem cell transplantation.

Acute myeloid leukemia (AML) is a type of leukemia that affects the myeloid cells in the bone marrow and blood. AML progresses quickly and can cause symptoms such as fatigue, shortness of breath, weight loss, and fever. Treatment for AML involves chemotherapy and sometimes stem cell transplantation.

Chronic lymphocytic leukemia (CLL) is a slow-growing cancer that affects the lymphocytes in the bone marrow and blood. CLL is most common in adults over the age of 55 and often has no symptoms in the early stages. As the disease progresses, symptoms may include fatigue, fever, weight loss, and swollen lymph nodes. Treatment for CLL may involve chemotherapy, immunotherapy, and targeted therapy.

Chronic myeloid leukemia (CML) is a type of leukemia that affects the myeloid cells in the bone marrow and blood. It is a slow-growing cancer that can progress to a more aggressive form. Symptoms of CML may include fatigue, night sweats, and abdominal pain. Treatment for CML may include chemotherapy, targeted therapy, and stem cell transplantation.

There are also less common types of leukemia, such as hairy cell leukemia, T-cell acute lymphoblastic leukemia, and myelodysplastic syndromes. These types of leukemia are characterized by the abnormal production of different types of white blood cells and may have unique symptoms and treatment options.

Leukemia is caused by changes in the DNA of blood-forming cells in the bone marrow. These changes may occur spontaneously or be caused by exposure to radiation, certain chemicals, or viruses. However, in many cases, the exact cause of leukemia is unknown.

The diagnosis of leukemia typically involves a series of tests, including blood tests, bone marrow biopsies, and imaging studies. These tests help doctors determine the type and stage of leukemia, which is important in developing a treatment plan.

Treatment for leukemia can vary depending on the type of the disease and how advanced it is. Some people may require a combination of treatments, such as chemotherapy, radiation therapy, and stem cell transplantation.

Chemotherapy is the most common treatment for leukemia and involves using drugs to kill cancer cells. Radiation therapy involves using high-energy radiation to kill cancer cells, while stem cell transplantation involves replacing damaged bone marrow with healthy cells from a donor.

Leukemia can be a challenging disease to manage, and many people require ongoing care and support. This may include regular check-ups, blood tests, and other monitoring to detect any signs of the disease returning.

leukemia is a type of cancer that affects the blood-forming cells in the bone marrow. It is a complex disease that can present in different forms, and while treatment options have improved over the years, it remains a serious and often life-threatening condition. Understanding the different types of leukemia and their symptoms is essential in order to diagnose, treat, and manage the disease. Ongoing research is needed to better understand the disease and develop new treatments that can help more people live longer, healthier lives.

Causes and Risk Factors

Leukemia is a type of cancer that affects the blood-forming cells in the bone marrow. It is a complex disease that can be caused by a variety of factors, including genetic mutations, environmental exposure, and lifestyle factors. Understanding the causes and risk factors for leukemia is essential in order to prevent and manage the disease.

Genetic mutations are a common cause of leukemia. These mutations can occur spontaneously or be inherited from a parent. Certain genetic mutations, such as the Philadelphia chromosome, are associated with specific types of leukemia, such as chronic myeloid leukemia (CML). Mutations in other genes, such as TP53 and ATM, are associated with an increased risk of developing acute lymphoblastic leukemia (ALL).

Exposure to certain environmental factors, such as radiation and chemicals, can also increase the risk of developing leukemia. High levels of ionizing radiation exposure, such as from nuclear accidents or medical treatments, have been linked to an increased risk of developing leukemia.

Exposure to certain chemicals, such as benzene and formaldehyde, can also increase the risk of developing leukemia.

Lifestyle factors can also contribute to the development of leukemia. Smoking has been linked to an increased risk of developing acute myeloid leukemia (AML), while obesity has been linked to an increased risk of developing chronic lymphocytic leukemia (CLL).

Certain medical conditions and treatments can also increase the risk of developing leukemia. For example, people with certain inherited disorders, such as Down syndrome and Fanconi anemia, are at an increased risk of developing leukemia. Chemotherapy and radiation therapy, while often used to treat cancer, can also increase the risk of developing leukemia later in life.

The symptoms of leukemia can vary depending on the type of the disease and how advanced it is. Common symptoms include fatigue, fever, night sweats, weight loss, and frequent infections. Other symptoms may include easy bruising or bleeding, pain or swelling in the abdomen, and swollen lymph nodes. However, many of these symptoms can be caused by other conditions, so it's important to see a doctor for a proper diagnosis.

Diagnosis of leukemia typically involves a series of tests, including blood tests, bone marrow biopsies, and imaging studies. These tests help doctors determine the type and stage of leukemia, which is important in developing a treatment plan.

Treatment for leukemia can vary depending on the type of the disease and how advanced it is. Some people may require a combination of treatments, such as chemotherapy, radiation therapy, and stem cell transplantation.

Chemotherapy is the most common treatment for leukemia and involves using drugs to kill cancer cells. Radiation therapy involves using high-energy radiation to kill cancer cells, while stem cell transplantation involves replacing damaged bone marrow with healthy cells from a donor.

Despite advances in treatment, leukemia can be a challenging disease to manage, and many people require ongoing care and support. This may include regular check-ups, blood tests, and other monitoring to detect any signs of the disease returning.

leukemia is a complex disease that can be caused by a variety of factors, including genetic mutations, environmental exposure, and lifestyle factors. Understanding the causes and risk factors for leukemia is essential in order to prevent and manage the disease. While treatment options have improved over the years, ongoing research is needed to better understand the disease and develop new treatments that can help more people live longer, healthier lives.

Epidemiology and Statistics

Leukemia is a type of cancer that affects the blood-forming cells in the bone marrow. It is a complex disease that can be seen across the world, with different patterns of incidence and mortality rates. Epidemiology and statistics play a vital role in understanding the prevalence, incidence, and mortality rates of leukemia, which can help inform public health policy and improve patient outcomes.

According to the World Health Organization (WHO), leukemia is the 11th most common cancer worldwide, with an estimated 437,000 new cases and 309,000 deaths in 2020. The incidence of leukemia varies by geography and age group. The highest incidence rates of leukemia are seen in North America and Europe, while the lowest rates are seen in Africa and Asia. In the United States, leukemia accounts for about 3.5% of all new cancer cases and 3.9% of all cancer deaths.

The incidence of leukemia also varies by age group. Acute lymphoblastic leukemia (ALL) is the most common type of leukemia in children, accounting for about 75% of all cases. The incidence of ALL peaks between the ages of 2 and 4 years and then declines until age 10. Acute myeloid leukemia (AML) is more common in adults, with the incidence increasing with age. Chronic lymphocytic leukemia (CLL) is most common in older adults, with the incidence increasing steadily with age.

Gender also plays a role in the incidence and mortality rates of leukemia. In general, males are more likely to develop leukemia than females. For example, the incidence rate of AML is 1.5 times higher in men than in women. However, the survival rates for males and females with leukemia are similar.

Several factors can increase the risk of developing leukemia. Exposure to ionizing radiation and certain chemicals, such as benzene and formaldehyde, have been linked to an increased risk of developing leukemia. People with certain genetic mutations, such as the Philadelphia chromosome, are also at an increased risk of developing leukemia.

The mortality rates of leukemia have improved over the years, with advances in treatment and supportive care. According to the American Cancer Society, the five-year relative survival rate for all types of leukemia combined has increased from 34% in the 1970s to 63% in recent years. However, the survival rates vary depending on the type and stage of leukemia, as well as other factors such as age and overall health.

epidemiology and statistics play a crucial role in understanding the prevalence, incidence, and mortality rates of leukemia. The incidence and mortality rates of leukemia vary by geography, age group, and gender. Understanding these patterns can help inform public health policy and improve patient outcomes. While the mortality rates of leukemia have improved over the years, ongoing research is needed to better understand the disease and develop new treatments that can help more people live longer, healthier lives.

Anatomy of Blood and Bone Marrow

Leukemia is a type of cancer that affects the blood-forming cells in the bone marrow. To understand how leukemia develops, it's important to have a basic understanding of the anatomy of the blood and bone marrow.

Blood is a vital fluid that circulates throughout the body, delivering oxygen and nutrients to tissues and organs and carrying waste products away. Blood is composed of different types of cells, including red blood cells, white blood cells, and platelets.

Red blood cells, or erythrocytes, are responsible for carrying oxygen from the lungs to the tissues and organs. They are produced in the bone marrow and have a lifespan of about 120 days.

White blood cells, or leukocytes, are a key component of the immune system, which helps the body fight infections and other diseases. There are several types of white blood cells, including lymphocytes, neutrophils, monocytes, eosinophils, and basophils.

Platelets, or thrombocytes, are small cells that play a vital role in blood clotting. They help stop bleeding by clumping together at the site of an injury and forming a plug.

The bone marrow is the soft, spongy tissue inside bones where blood cells are produced. It is a complex organ that contains different types of cells, including hematopoietic stem cells, which are responsible for producing all types of blood cells.

Hematopoietic stem cells are unique cells that have the ability to differentiate into different types of blood cells. They can give rise to myeloid cells, which include red blood cells, platelets, and several types of white blood cells, as well as lymphoid cells, which include T cells, B cells, and natural killer cells.

In healthy individuals, the production of blood cells in the bone marrow is tightly regulated. However, in leukemia, the production of blood cells becomes abnormal, leading to the overproduction of immature or damaged white blood cells.

There are several types of leukemia, which can be classified based on how quickly the disease progresses and the type of white blood cells affected. Acute leukemias, such as acute lymphoblastic leukemia (ALL) and acute myeloid leukemia (AML), progress quickly and require immediate treatment. Chronic leukemias, such as chronic lymphocytic leukemia (CLL) and chronic myeloid leukemia (CML), progress more slowly and may not require immediate treatment.

In leukemia, the abnormal production of white blood cells can lead to a variety of symptoms, including fatigue, fever, weight loss, and frequent infections. Other symptoms may include easy bruising or bleeding, pain or swelling in the abdomen, and swollen lymph nodes.

Diagnosis of leukemia typically involves a series of tests, including blood tests, bone marrow biopsies, and imaging studies. These tests help doctors determine the type and stage of leukemia, which is important in developing a treatment plan.

Treatment for leukemia can vary depending on the type of the disease and how advanced it is. Some people may require a combination of treatments, such as chemotherapy, radiation therapy, and stem cell transplantation.

understanding the anatomy of blood and bone marrow is essential in order to understand how leukemia develops and how it affects the body. Leukemia is a complex disease that can present in different forms, and while treatment options have improved over the years, it remains a serious and often life-threatening condition. Ongoing research is needed to better understand the disease and develop new treatments that can help more people live longer, healthier lives.

Components of Blood

Blood is a vital fluid that circulates throughout the body, delivering oxygen and nutrients to tissues and organs and carrying waste products away. It is composed of different components, including red blood cells, white blood cells, platelets, and plasma. Understanding the components of blood is essential in order to understand how leukemia develops and how it affects the body.

Red blood cells, or erythrocytes, are responsible for carrying oxygen from the lungs to the tissues and organs. They contain hemoglobin, a protein that binds to oxygen and helps transport it throughout the body. Red blood cells are produced in the bone marrow and have a lifespan of about 120 days.

White blood cells, or leukocytes, are a key component of the immune system, which helps the body fight infections and other diseases. There are several types of white blood cells, including lymphocytes, neutrophils, monocytes, eosinophils, and basophils. Each type of white blood cell plays a specific role in the immune system.

1. Lymphocytes are a type of white blood cell that play a critical role in the immune response. There are two main types of lymphocytes: B cells and T cells. B cells produce antibodies, which help to identify and neutralize

foreign substances in the body. T cells, on the other hand, play a key role in recognizing and destroying infected or cancerous cells.

Neutrophils are the most common type of white blood cell, and they play a vital role in fighting bacterial infections. They are responsible for engulfing and destroying bacteria and other foreign substances in the body.

Monocytes are another type of white blood cell that play a key role in the immune response. They are responsible for engulfing and destroying foreign substances, such as bacteria and viruses.

Eosinophils and basophils are less common types of white blood cells that play a role in the immune response. Eosinophils are involved in fighting parasitic infections and allergic reactions, while basophils are involved in allergic reactions.

Platelets, or thrombocytes, are small cells that play a vital role in blood clotting. They help stop bleeding by clumping together at the site of an injury and forming a plug.

Plasma is the liquid component of blood, and it makes up about 55% of the total volume of blood. Plasma is composed of water, electrolytes, and a variety of proteins, including albumin, globulin, and fibrinogen. These proteins help regulate blood pressure, maintain the balance of fluids in the body, and assist in blood clotting.

Leukemia is a type of cancer that affects the blood-forming cells in the bone marrow. In leukemia, the abnormal production of white blood cells can lead to a variety of symptoms, including fatigue, fever, weight loss, and frequent infections. Other symptoms may include easy bruising or bleeding, pain or swelling in the abdomen, and swollen lymph nodes.

The diagnosis of leukemia typically involves a series of tests, including blood tests, bone marrow biopsies, and imaging studies. These tests help doctors determine the type and stage of leukemia, which is important in developing a treatment plan.

Treatment for leukemia can vary depending on the type of the disease and how advanced it is. Some people may require a combination of treatments, such as chemotherapy, radiation therapy, and stem cell transplantation.

understanding the components of blood is essential in order to understand how leukemia develops and how it affects the body. Leukemia is a complex disease that can present in different forms, and while treatment options have improved over the years, it remains a serious and often life-threatening condition. Ongoing research is needed to better understand the disease and develop new treatments that can help more people live longer, healthier lives.

Bone Marrow Structure and Function

Bone marrow is a spongy tissue located in the hollow cavities of bones, and it is responsible for the production of blood cells. The structure and function of bone marrow are critical for understanding how leukemia develops and how it affects the body.

The bone marrow contains different types of cells, including hematopoietic stem cells (HSCs), stromal cells, and endothelial cells. HSCs are responsible for the production of all blood cells, including red blood cells, white blood cells, and platelets. Stromal cells provide support to the HSCs and help regulate their function, while endothelial cells line the blood vessels in the bone marrow.

HSCs are unique cells that have the ability to differentiate into different types of blood cells. They can give rise to myeloid cells, which include red blood cells, platelets, and several types of white blood cells, as well as lymphoid cells, which include T cells, B cells, and natural killer cells.

The process of blood cell production, or hematopoiesis, occurs in the bone marrow through a complex process involving different cell types and signaling molecules. The process begins with the HSCs, which differentiate into different types of progenitor cells, including erythroblasts, megakaryoblasts, and myeloblasts.

Erythroblasts are the progenitor cells that give rise to red blood cells, while megakaryoblasts give rise to platelets. Myeloblasts, on the other hand, give rise to different types of white blood cells, including neutrophils, monocytes, eosinophils, and basophils.

In leukemia, the production of blood cells becomes abnormal, leading to the overproduction of immature or damaged white blood cells. There are several types of leukemia, which can be classified based on how quickly the disease progresses and the type of white blood cells affected.

Acute leukemias, such as acute lymphoblastic leukemia (ALL) and acute myeloid leukemia (AML), progress quickly and require immediate treatment. Chronic leukemias, such as chronic lymphocytic leukemia (CLL) and chronic myeloid leukemia (CML), progress more slowly and may not require immediate treatment.

The diagnosis of leukemia typically involves a series of tests, including blood tests, bone marrow biopsies, and imaging studies. These tests help doctors determine the type and stage of leukemia, which is important in developing a treatment plan.

Treatment for leukemia can vary depending on the type of the disease and how advanced it is. Some people may require a combination of treatments, such as chemotherapy, radiation therapy, and stem cell transplantation.

Stem cell transplantation is a procedure that involves replacing the damaged bone marrow with healthy HSCs from a donor. The procedure can be used to treat leukemia and other blood disorders, and it involves destroying the patient's own bone marrow using chemotherapy or radiation therapy before transplanting the donor cells.

bone marrow is a vital tissue that plays a critical role in the production of blood cells. Understanding the structure and function of bone marrow is essential in order to understand how leukemia develops and how it affects the body. Leukemia is a complex disease that can present in different forms, and while treatment options have improved over the years, it remains a serious and often life-threatening condition. Ongoing research is needed to better understand the disease and develop new treatments that can help more people live longer, healthier lives.

Hematopoiesis

Hematopoiesis is the process of blood cell production, which occurs in the bone marrow. The process is tightly regulated and involves the differentiation of hematopoietic stem cells (HSCs) into different types of blood cells. Understanding hematopoiesis is essential for understanding how leukemia develops and how it affects the body.

Hematopoietic stem cells are unique cells that have the ability to differentiate into different types of blood cells. They can give rise to myeloid cells, which include red blood cells, platelets, and several types of white blood cells, as well as lymphoid cells, which include T cells, B cells, and natural killer cells.

The process of hematopoiesis involves several steps, including proliferation, differentiation, and maturation. During proliferation, HSCs undergo rapid cell division to produce a pool of progenitor cells, which can differentiate into different types of blood cells.

Differentiation involves the process of becoming a specific type of blood cell. For example, erythroblasts differentiate into red blood cells, while megakaryoblasts differentiate into platelets. Myeloblasts differentiate into different types of white blood cells, including neutrophils, monocytes, eosinophils, and basophils.

Maturation is the final step in the process, and it involves the development of fully functional blood cells. Mature blood cells are released into the bloodstream and are able to perform their specific functions, such as carrying oxygen or fighting infections.

Leukemia is a type of cancer that affects the blood-forming cells in the bone marrow. In leukemia, the production of blood cells becomes abnormal, leading to the overproduction of immature or damaged white blood cells. There are several types of leukemia, which can be classified based on how quickly the disease progresses and the type of white blood cells affected.

Acute leukemias, such as acute lymphoblastic leukemia (ALL) and acute myeloid leukemia (AML), progress quickly and require immediate treatment. Chronic leukemias, such as chronic lymphocytic leukemia (CLL) and chronic myeloid leukemia (CML), progress more slowly and may not require immediate treatment.

The diagnosis of leukemia typically involves a series of tests, including blood tests, bone marrow biopsies, and imaging studies. These tests help doctors determine the type and stage of leukemia, which is important in developing a treatment plan.

Treatment for leukemia can vary depending on the type of the disease and how advanced it is. Some people may require a combination of treatments, such as chemotherapy, radiation therapy, and stem cell transplantation.

Stem cell transplantation is a procedure that involves replacing the damaged bone marrow with healthy HSCs from a donor. The procedure can be used to treat leukemia and other blood disorders, and it involves destroying the patient's own bone marrow using chemotherapy or radiation therapy before transplanting the donor cells.

hematopoiesis is a complex process that involves the production of all types of blood cells. Understanding hematopoiesis is essential for understanding how leukemia develops and how it affects the body. Leukemia is a complex disease that can present in different forms, and while treatment options have improved over the years, it remains a serious and often life-threatening condition. Ongoing research is needed to better understand the disease and develop new treatments that can help more people live longer, healthier lives.

Pathophysiology of Leukemia

Leukemia is a type of cancer that affects the blood-forming cells in the bone marrow. The pathophysiology of leukemia involves the abnormal production and function of white blood cells, which can lead to a variety of symptoms and complications.

In a healthy individual, hematopoietic stem cells (HSCs) differentiate into different types of blood cells, including red blood cells, white blood cells, and platelets. In leukemia, the production of white blood cells becomes abnormal, leading to the overproduction of immature or damaged cells.

There are several types of leukemia, which can be classified based on how quickly the disease progresses and the type of white blood cells affected. Acute leukemias, such as acute lymphoblastic leukemia (ALL) and acute myeloid leukemia (AML), progress quickly and require immediate treatment. Chronic leukemias, such as chronic lymphocytic leukemia (CLL) and chronic myeloid leukemia (CML), progress more slowly and may not require immediate treatment.

The abnormal white blood cells in leukemia can interfere with the production of other types of blood cells, leading to a variety of symptoms and complications. For example, the overproduction of white blood cells can lead to a decrease in the number of red blood cells, which can cause fatigue, weakness, and shortness of breath.

The abnormal white blood cells can also interfere with the production of platelets, which can lead to bleeding and bruising. In addition, the abnormal white blood cells can accumulate in various organs, such as the liver and spleen, causing enlargement and dysfunction of these organs.

The pathophysiology of leukemia involves several genetic and environmental factors that can contribute to the development of the disease. Genetic mutations in the HSCs can disrupt the normal process of differentiation and lead to the overproduction of white blood cells. Exposure to certain chemicals, such as benzene, and radiation can also increase the risk of developing leukemia.

The diagnosis of leukemia typically involves a series of tests, including blood tests, bone marrow biopsies, and imaging studies. These tests help doctors determine the type and stage of leukemia, which is important in developing a treatment plan.

Treatment for leukemia can vary depending on the type of the disease and how advanced it is. Some people may require a combination of treatments, such as chemotherapy, radiation therapy, and stem cell transplantation.

Chemotherapy involves the use of drugs to kill cancer cells, while radiation therapy uses high-energy radiation to kill cancer cells. Stem cell transplantation involves replacing the damaged bone marrow with healthy HSCs from a donor.

the pathophysiology of leukemia involves the abnormal production and function of white blood cells, which can lead to a variety of symptoms and complications. The development of leukemia involves several genetic and environmental factors, and the diagnosis and treatment of the disease requires a multidisciplinary approach. Ongoing research is needed to better understand the disease and develop new treatments that can help more people live longer, healthier lives.

Genetic and Molecular Abnormalities

Leukemia is a type of cancer that affects the blood-forming cells in the bone marrow. The development of leukemia is often associated with genetic and molecular abnormalities that can disrupt the normal process of hematopoiesis and lead to the overproduction of white blood cells.

Genetic and molecular abnormalities in leukemia can involve changes in the DNA or RNA of blood-forming cells. These changes can occur spontaneously or as a result of exposure to certain chemicals or radiation. Some of the most common genetic and molecular abnormalities associated with leukemia include:

1. Chromosomal abnormalities: Changes in the number or structure of chromosomes can disrupt the normal process of hematopoiesis and lead

to the overproduction of white blood cells. For example, the Philadelphia chromosome, which is present in most cases of chronic myeloid leukemia (CML), results from a translocation between chromosomes 9 and 22, leading to the formation of a fusion gene called BCR-ABL1.

2. Gene mutations: Mutations in genes that regulate the growth and differentiation of blood-forming cells can also contribute to the development of leukemia. For example, mutations in the FLT3 gene are common in acute myeloid leukemia (AML) and can lead to the overproduction of white blood cells.

3. Epigenetic changes: Epigenetic changes involve modifications to the DNA that do not affect the actual sequence of the DNA, but can still have an impact on gene expression. For example, changes in the methylation status of certain genes can lead to the overproduction of white blood cells in leukemia.

4. RNA abnormalities: Changes in the expression or function of RNA molecules can also contribute to the development of leukemia. For example, aberrant splicing of RNA molecules can lead to the overproduction of white blood cells in leukemia.

The identification of genetic and molecular abnormalities in leukemia has led to the development of targeted therapies that can specifically inhibit or target these abnormalities. For example, drugs such as imatinib and dasatinib target the BCR-ABL1 fusion gene in CML, while drugs such as midostaurin and gilteritinib target the FLT3 gene in AML.

In addition to targeted therapies, genetic and molecular abnormalities in leukemia can also be used to monitor the response to treatment and to predict the likelihood of relapse. For example, the detection of minimal residual disease (MRD), which involves the detection of residual cancer cells after treatment, can help predict the likelihood of relapse and guide treatment decisions.

genetic and molecular abnormalities play a critical role in the development and progression of leukemia. The identification of these abnormalities has led to the development of targeted therapies and improved the ability to monitor response to treatment and predict the likelihood of relapse. Ongoing research is needed to better understand the role of these abnormalities in leukemia and to develop new treatments that can help more people live longer, healthier lives.

Leukemic Cell Development

Leukemia is a type of cancer that affects the blood-forming cells in the bone marrow. The development of leukemia is often associated with abnormalities in the development of leukemic cells, which can lead to the overproduction of immature or damaged white blood cells.

Leukemic cells develop from hematopoietic stem cells (HSCs) that undergo a series of genetic and molecular changes that disrupt the normal process of hematopoiesis. These changes can involve alterations in the DNA or RNA of blood-forming cells, as well as changes in the microenvironment of the bone marrow.

The development of leukemic cells can be divided into several stages, including initiation, promotion, and progression. During the initiation phase, genetic or environmental factors can trigger changes in the DNA or RNA of HSCs, leading to the development of pre-leukemic cells.

During the promotion phase, pre-leukemic cells undergo additional genetic and molecular changes that increase their proliferation and survival. These changes can involve the activation of oncogenes or the inactivation of tumor suppressor genes, as well as changes in the microenvironment of the bone marrow.

During the progression phase, pre-leukemic cells become fully transformed into leukemic cells, which can overproduce immature or damaged white blood cells. The development of leukemic cells can also be influenced by the presence of mutations or abnormalities in other genes, such as those involved in DNA repair or cell cycle regulation.

The development of leukemic cells is a complex process that involves multiple genetic and environmental factors. The identification of these factors has led to the development of targeted therapies that can specifically inhibit or target the abnormalities in leukemic cells.

For example, drugs such as imatinib and dasatinib target the BCR-ABL1 fusion gene in chronic myeloid leukemia (CML), while drugs such as midostaurin and gilteritinib target the FLT3 gene in acute myeloid leukemia (AML).

In addition to targeted therapies, the development of leukemic cells can also be monitored using techniques such as flow cytometry, which can identify the presence of leukemic cells in the blood or bone marrow. The detection of minimal residual disease (MRD), which involves the detection of residual cancer cells after treatment, can also help predict the likelihood of relapse and guide treatment decisions.

the development of leukemic cells is a complex process that involves multiple genetic and environmental factors. Understanding the mechanisms underlying the development of leukemic cells is essential for the development of targeted therapies and improved monitoring of treatment response. Ongoing research is needed to better understand the role of these factors in leukemia and to develop new treatments that can help more people live longer, healthier lives.

Effects on Normal Blood Cells

Leukemia is a type of cancer that affects the blood-forming cells in the bone marrow. The abnormal production and function of white blood cells in leukemia can have a significant impact on the normal blood cells in the body, leading to a variety of symptoms and complications.

Red blood cells, white blood cells, and platelets are the three main types of blood cells in the body, each with its own important function. The abnormal production and function of white blood cells in leukemia can interfere with the production and function of other types of blood cells.

Red blood cells are responsible for carrying oxygen from the lungs to the rest of the body. In leukemia, the overproduction of white blood cells can lead to a decrease in the number of red blood cells, which can cause anemia. Anemia can cause fatigue, weakness, shortness of breath, and pale skin.

White blood cells are responsible for fighting infections and diseases. In leukemia, the overproduction of abnormal white blood cells can interfere with the production and function of normal white blood cells, making it more difficult for the body to fight infections. This can lead to an increased risk of infections, such as pneumonia or sepsis.

Platelets are responsible for helping the blood clot, which is important in preventing excessive bleeding. In leukemia, the abnormal white blood cells can interfere with the production and function of platelets, leading to a decreased ability of the blood to clot. This can cause bleeding and bruising, such as nosebleeds, bleeding gums, or excessive bruising.

In addition to the effects on normal blood cells, leukemia can also cause enlargement and dysfunction of organs such as the liver and spleen. This can lead to abdominal pain, fullness, and discomfort.

The effects on normal blood cells in leukemia can be managed through a variety of treatments, depending on the type and stage of the disease. For example, blood transfusions can be used to increase the number of red blood cells or platelets in the body. Medications can also be used to boost the production of normal white blood cells or to prevent infections.

In some cases, chemotherapy, radiation therapy, or stem cell transplantation may be necessary to treat the underlying leukemia and restore the normal production and function of blood cells. The type and duration of treatment can vary depending on the individual case and response to treatment.

leukemia can have a significant impact on the normal blood cells in the body, leading to a variety of symptoms and complications. The effects on normal blood cells can be managed through a variety of treatments, depending on the type and stage of the disease. Ongoing research is needed to better understand the effects of leukemia on normal blood cells and to develop new treatments that can help more people live longer, healthier lives.

Signs and Symptoms

Leukemia is a type of cancer that affects the blood-forming cells in the bone marrow. The signs and symptoms of leukemia can vary depending on the type and stage of the disease. Some people with leukemia may have no symptoms at all, while others may experience a range of symptoms that can impact their daily lives.

The signs and symptoms of leukemia can be divided into several categories, including those related to the abnormal production and function of white blood cells, anemia, and bleeding and bruising.

Symptoms related to the abnormal production and function of white blood cells:

Fatigue

Weakness

Fever or chills

Night sweats

Infections that do not go away or keep coming back

Swollen lymph nodes

Abdominal discomfort or pain

Bone or joint pain

Loss of appetite or weight loss

Symptoms related to anemia:

Fatigue

Weakness

Shortness of breath

Pale skin

Symptoms related to bleeding and bruising:

Easy bruising or bleeding

Petechiae (small red or purple spots on the skin)

Nosebleeds

Bleeding gums

Heavy or prolonged menstrual periods

In addition to these symptoms, some people with leukemia may also experience other nonspecific symptoms, such as headaches, vision changes, or dizziness.

The signs and symptoms of leukemia can be similar to those of other conditions, making diagnosis difficult. If you experience any of these symptoms, it is important to see a doctor for an evaluation. Early diagnosis and treatment of leukemia can improve the chances of a successful outcome.

Diagnosis of leukemia typically involves a series of tests, including blood tests, bone marrow biopsies, and imaging studies. These tests help doctors determine the type and stage of leukemia, which is important in developing a treatment plan.

Treatment for leukemia can vary depending on the type and stage of the disease. Some people may require a combination of treatments, such as chemotherapy, radiation therapy, and stem cell transplantation.

Chemotherapy involves the use of drugs to kill cancer cells, while radiation therapy uses high-energy radiation to kill cancer cells. Stem cell transplantation involves replacing the damaged bone marrow with healthy hematopoietic stem cells from a donor.

leukemia can cause a range of signs and symptoms that can impact a person's daily life. These symptoms can be related to the abnormal production and function of white blood cells, anemia, or bleeding and bruising. Early diagnosis and treatment of leukemia is important in improving the chances of a successful outcome. If you experience any of these symptoms, it is important to see a doctor for an evaluation.

General Symptoms

Leukemia is a type of cancer that affects the blood-forming cells in the bone marrow. The disease can cause a range of symptoms that can impact a person's daily life. Some symptoms are specific to leukemia, while others are more general and can be seen in other conditions as well.

General symptoms of leukemia can include fatigue, weakness, fever, and weight loss. These symptoms are often nonspecific and can be caused by a variety of conditions, which can make diagnosis challenging. However, if these symptoms are persistent or severe, it is important to see a doctor for evaluation.

Fatigue and weakness are common symptoms in leukemia. The abnormal production and function of white blood cells can cause fatigue and weakness by interfering with the body's ability to fight infections and transport oxygen to the tissues. Fatigue and weakness can be persistent and impact a person's ability to perform daily activities.

Fever is another common symptom in leukemia. The overproduction of abnormal white blood cells can cause fever by triggering an immune response in the body. Fever can be a sign of infection, which can be a complication of leukemia.

Weight loss is another symptom that can be seen in leukemia. The overproduction of abnormal white blood cells can cause weight loss by increasing the body's metabolic rate and decreasing appetite. Weight loss can be a persistent symptom that can impact a person's overall health.

In addition to these general symptoms, leukemia can cause specific symptoms depending on the type and stage of the disease. For example, acute lymphoblastic leukemia (ALL) can cause bone pain and joint pain, while chronic lymphocytic leukemia (CLL) can cause enlarged lymph nodes and spleen.

Acute myeloid leukemia (AML) can cause fever, fatigue, and bleeding and bruising. Acute promyelocytic leukemia (APL) can cause bleeding and clotting problems, while hairy cell leukemia (HCL) can cause infections, fatigue, and enlarged spleen.

Diagnosis of leukemia typically involves a series of tests, including blood tests, bone marrow biopsies, and imaging studies. These tests help doctors determine the type and stage of leukemia, which is important in developing a treatment plan.

Treatment for leukemia can vary depending on the type and stage of the disease. Some people may require a combination of treatments, such as chemotherapy, radiation therapy, and stem cell transplantation.

Chemotherapy involves the use of drugs to kill cancer cells, while radiation therapy uses high-energy radiation to kill cancer cells. Stem cell transplantation involves replacing the damaged bone marrow with healthy hematopoietic stem cells from a donor.

leukemia can cause a range of general symptoms, such as fatigue, weakness, fever, and weight loss, as well as specific symptoms depending on the type and stage of the disease. If these symptoms are persistent or severe, it is important to see a doctor for evaluation. Early diagnosis and treatment of leukemia is important in improving the chances of a successful outcome.

Organ-Specific Manifestations

Leukemia is a type of cancer that affects the blood-forming cells in the bone marrow. The disease can cause a range of symptoms and complications that can impact various organs and systems in the body. Organ-specific manifestations of leukemia can vary depending on the type and stage of the disease.

Some of the common organ-specific manifestations of leukemia are as follows:

Central Nervous System (CNS) Manifestations:

Leukemia can affect the CNS by invading the brain and spinal cord. This can cause symptoms such as headaches, seizures, confusion, and speech difficulties. Acute lymphoblastic leukemia (ALL) and acute myeloid leukemia (AML) are more likely to affect the CNS.

Respiratory System Manifestations:

Leukemia can cause respiratory symptoms such as cough, shortness of breath, and chest pain. This can occur due to leukemic cells infiltrating the lungs or due to lung infections. Acute monocytic leukemia (AML-M5) is more likely to affect the lungs.

Gastrointestinal System Manifestations:

Leukemia can affect the gastrointestinal system by causing abdominal pain, nausea, vomiting, and diarrhea. This can occur due to leukemic cells infiltrating the intestines or due to infections. Acute monocytic leukemia (AML-M5) and chronic myeloid leukemia (CML) are more likely to affect the gastrointestinal system.

Renal System Manifestations:

Leukemia can cause renal symptoms such as proteinuria, hematuria, and renal failure. This can occur due to leukemic cells infiltrating the kidneys or due to infections. Acute myeloid leukemia (AML) and chronic lymphocytic leukemia (CLL) are more likely to affect the renal system.

Hepatic System Manifestations:

Leukemia can cause hepatic symptoms such as hepatomegaly, jaundice, and elevated liver enzymes. This can occur due to leukemic cells infiltrating the liver or due to infections. Acute monocytic leukemia (AML-M5) and chronic lymphocytic leukemia (CLL) are more likely to affect the hepatic system.

Musculoskeletal System Manifestations:

Leukemia can cause musculoskeletal symptoms such as bone pain, joint pain, and osteoporosis. This can occur due to leukemic cells infiltrating the bones or due to osteoporosis caused by chemotherapy. Acute lymphoblastic leukemia (ALL) and acute myeloid leukemia (AML) are more likely to affect the musculoskeletal system.

Diagnosis of leukemia typically involves a series of tests, including blood tests, bone marrow biopsies, and imaging studies. These tests help doctors determine the type and stage of leukemia, which is important in developing a treatment plan.

Treatment for leukemia can vary depending on the type and stage of the disease. Some people may require a combination of treatments, such as chemotherapy, radiation therapy, and stem cell transplantation.

Chemotherapy involves the use of drugs to kill cancer cells, while radiation therapy uses high-energy radiation to kill cancer cells. Stem cell transplantation involves replacing the damaged bone marrow with healthy hematopoietic stem cells from a donor.

leukemia can cause a range of organ-specific manifestations depending on the type and stage of the disease. These manifestations can impact various organs and systems in the body, such as the central nervous system, respiratory system, gastrointestinal system, renal system, hepatic system, and musculoskeletal system. If you experience any of these symptoms, it is important to see a doctor for evaluation. Early diagnosis and treatment of leukemia is important in improving the chances of a successful outcome.

Complications

Leukemia is a type of cancer that affects the blood-forming cells in the bone marrow. The disease can cause a range of symptoms and complications that can impact various organs and systems in the body. Complications of leukemia can vary depending on the type and stage of the disease.

Some of the common complications of leukemia are as follows:

Infections:

Leukemia can weaken the immune system, making people more susceptible to infections. These infections can be bacterial, viral, or fungal in nature and can occur anywhere in the body. Infections can cause symptoms such as fever, chills, cough, and shortness of breath.

Anemia:

Leukemia can cause a reduction in red blood cells, leading to anemia. Anemia can cause symptoms such as fatigue, weakness, shortness of breath, and pale skin. Severe anemia can lead to complications such as heart failure.

Bleeding and Bruising:

Leukemia can cause a reduction in platelets, leading to bleeding and bruising. Platelets are essential for blood clotting, and their reduction can cause symptoms such as nosebleeds, bleeding gums, and easy bruising. Severe bleeding can lead to life-threatening complications.

Tumor Lysis Syndrome:

Leukemia treatment can cause the rapid breakdown of cancer cells, releasing large amounts of waste products into the bloodstream. This can lead to tumor lysis syndrome, which can cause symptoms such as kidney failure, electrolyte imbalances, and cardiac arrhythmias.

Organ Failure:

Leukemia can infiltrate various organs in the body, leading to organ failure. This can occur due to leukemic cells invading the organs or due to complications such as infections and bleeding. Organ failure can cause symptoms such as abdominal pain, jaundice, and renal failure.

Neurological Complications:

Leukemia can cause neurological complications such as headaches, seizures, and confusion. This can occur due to leukemic cells invading the brain or due to complications such as infections and bleeding.

Secondary Cancers:

Leukemia treatment can increase the risk of developing secondary cancers such as lymphoma, solid tumors, and myelodysplastic syndromes. These cancers can occur years after the initial leukemia treatment.

Diagnosis of leukemia typically involves a series of tests, including blood tests, bone marrow biopsies, and imaging studies. These tests help doctors determine the type and stage of leukemia, which is important in developing a treatment plan.

Treatment for leukemia can vary depending on the type and stage of the disease. Some people may require a combination of treatments, such as chemotherapy, radiation therapy, and stem cell transplantation.

Chemotherapy involves the use of drugs to kill cancer cells, while radiation therapy uses high-energy radiation to kill cancer cells. Stem cell transplantation involves replacing the damaged bone marrow with healthy hematopoietic stem cells from a donor.

leukemia can cause a range of complications depending on the type and stage of the disease. These complications can impact various organs and systems in the body and can lead to life-threatening complications. If you experience any of these symptoms or complications, it is important to see a doctor for evaluation. Early diagnosis and treatment of leukemia is important in improving the chances of a successful outcome.

Chapter Two

The different types of Leukemia

Leukemia is a type of cancer that affects the blood and bone marrow, and there are several different types of Leukemia. Here are some of the main types:

Acute Lymphoblastic Leukemia (ALL): This is the most common type of Leukemia in young children, but it can also occur in adults. ALL affects the lymphocytes, which are a type of white blood cell. Symptoms of ALL can include fatigue, fever, infections, bruising, and bleeding.

Acute Myeloid Leukemia (AML): AML is a type of Leukemia that affects the myeloid cells, which are responsible for producing red blood cells, white blood cells, and platelets. Symptoms of AML can include fatigue, infections, bruising, and bleeding.

Chronic Lymphocytic Leukemia (CLL): CLL is a type of Leukemia that affects the lymphocytes, and it is more common in older adults. Symptoms of CLL can include fatigue, fever, infections, and swollen lymph nodes.

Chronic Myeloid Leukemia (CML): CML is a type of Leukemia that affects the myeloid cells, and it is more common in adults. Symptoms of CML can include fatigue, fever, infections, and abdominal swelling.

Hairy Cell Leukemia (HCL): HCL is a rare type of Leukemia that affects the B-cells, which are a type of white blood cell. Symptoms of HCL can include fatigue, infections, and weakness.

Juvenile Myelomonocytic Leukemia (JMML): JMML is a rare type of Leukemia that usually affects children under the age of four. It is a chronic form of Leukemia that affects the myeloid cells. Symptoms of JMML can include infections, bruising, and bleeding.

Each type of Leukemia has different symptoms, treatment options, and outcomes. It's important to consult with a medical professional if you suspect you may have Leukemia or if you have been diagnosed with the disease.

Acute

L

ymphocytic

Leukemia

Acute lymphocytic Leukemia, also known as acute lymphoblastic Leukemia (ALL), is a type of blood cancer that affects the white blood cells in the bone marrow. It is the most common type of childhood Leukemia, but it can also affect adults.

In ALL, the bone marrow produces an excessive number of immature white blood cells, called lymphoblasts. These abnormal cells grow rapidly and accumulate in the bone marrow, preventing the normal production of red blood cells, white blood cells, and platelets. As a result, people with ALL may experience symptoms such as fatigue, weakness, infections, bleeding, and bruising.

The exact cause of ALL is not known, but certain risk factors have been identified, such as genetic predisposition, exposure to high doses of radiation, certain viral infections, and certain chemicals. However, most cases of ALL occur without any known risk factors.

ALL is diagnosed through a combination of physical examination, blood tests, and bone marrow biopsy. Treatment for ALL typically involves chemotherapy, radiation therapy, and sometimes stem cell transplantation. With appropriate treatment, many people with ALL can achieve remission, but long-term survival rates vary depending on the subtype of ALL and other factors.

Acute

M

yelogenous

Leukemia

(AML)

Acute myelogenous Leukemia (AML) is a type of cancer that starts in the bone marrow. AML is a type of Leukemia that affects the myeloid cells, which are responsible for producing red blood cells, white blood cells, and platelets. In AML, the myeloid cells do not mature into healthy blood cells, but instead grow uncontrollably, crowding out healthy cells in the bone marrow.

AML can affect people of any age, but it is more common in older adults. It can develop rapidly, and symptoms may appear suddenly. Symptoms of AML may include fatigue, shortness of breath, pale skin, frequent infections, easy bruising or bleeding, and bone pain.

The causes of AML are not fully understood, but certain factors may increase the risk of developing the disease. These risk factors may include exposure to certain chemicals or radiation, certain genetic disorders, and previous chemotherapy or radiation therapy.

Treatment for AML may involve chemotherapy, radiation therapy, and stem cell transplant. The specific treatment plan may depend on the subtype of AML, the age and health of the patient, and other factors. With early diagnosis and appropriate treatment, some patients with AML may achieve long-term remission. However, AML can be a life-threatening condition, and some cases may be difficult to treat.

Chronic Lymphocytic Leukemia (CLL)

Chronic lymphocytic Leukemia (CLL) is a type of Leukemia that affects the white blood cells in the body. It is a slow-growing cancer that develops in the bone marrow, where blood cells are produced. In CLL, the body produces too many abnormal lymphocytes, a type of white blood cell that helps the body fight infections. These abnormal cells do not function properly and may accumulate in the lymph nodes and other parts of the body.

CLL is the most common type of Leukemia in adults, with a higher incidence in older people. The exact causes of CLL are not fully understood, but it is believed to be related to genetic and environmental factors. CLL can be diagnosed through a blood test and a bone marrow biopsy.

The symptoms of CLL can vary depending on the stage of the disease, but may include fatigue, swollen lymph nodes, night sweats, unexplained weight loss, and frequent infections. Treatment options for CLL may include chemotherapy, radiation therapy, targeted therapy, and stem cell transplantation. The choice of treatment depends on the individual patient's health, age, and the stage of the disease.

With proper treatment, many people with CLL can manage the disease and live normal lives. However, because CLL is a chronic condition, people with CLL require ongoing monitoring and care to manage their symptoms and reduce the risk of complications.

Chronic

M

yelogenous

Leukemia

(CML)

Chronic myelogenous Leukemia (CML) is a type of blood cancer that affects the bone marrow, the spongy tissue inside the bones where blood cells are produced. In CML, the bone marrow produces too many immature white blood cells called myeloid cells, which accumulate in the bone marrow and interfere with the production of other blood cells.

CML is a chronic Leukemia, meaning it tends to progress slowly over time, often without causing any symptoms in the early stages. However, as the number of myeloid cells increases, they can eventually spill out of the bone marrow and into the bloodstream, causing a range of symptoms such as fatigue, weakness, and anemia.

CML is caused by a genetic mutation that affects a specific gene called the Philadelphia chromosome, which is present in more than 95% of patients with CML. This genetic mutation causes the bone marrow cells to produce an abnormal protein that drives the uncontrolled growth of myeloid cells.

Treatment for CML typically involves medications called tyrosine kinase inhibitors (TKIs) that target the abnormal protein produced by the Philadelphia chromosome. In some cases, a bone marrow or stem cell transplant may be necessary to replace the diseased bone marrow with healthy donor cells.

H

airy

C

ell

Leukemia

Hairy cell Leukemia is a rare type of chronic lymphocytic Leukemia (CLL) that gets its name from the unusual appearance of the cancer cells under a microscope. The cells look "hairy" due to fine projections on their surface.

Hairy cell Leukemia develops when the body produces too many abnormal B cells, a type of white blood cell that fights infection. The cancerous B cells accumulate in the bone marrow and interfere with the production of healthy blood cells, including red blood cells and platelets.

Hairy cell Leukemia is typically a slow-growing cancer, and many people with the disease have no symptoms in the early stages. However, as the disease progresses, symptoms may include fatigue, weakness, infections, fever, and enlarged spleen and liver.

Treatment options for hairy cell Leukemia include chemotherapy, immunotherapy, and targeted therapy. In some cases, a bone marrow or stem cell transplant may be recommended. With early diagnosis and proper treatment, many people with hairy cell Leukemia are able to achieve remission and live long, healthy lives.

M

yelodysplastic

S

yndromes

Myelodysplastic syndromes, also known as MDS, are a group of disorders that affect the bone marrow and blood cells. In MDS, the bone marrow produces immature or abnormal blood cells that don't function properly. These cells can't do their job, which is to fight off infection and transport oxygen throughout the body.

MDS can be caused by a number of factors, including exposure to certain chemicals, radiation, or chemotherapy. It can also be caused by genetic mutations or by a weakened immune system. MDS is more common in older adults, and men are more likely to develop the disease than women.

The symptoms of MDS can vary depending on the type and severity of the disease, but they can include fatigue, weakness, shortness of breath, and an increased risk of infection. Some people with MDS may not have any symptoms at all.

There is no cure for MDS, but treatment can help manage the symptoms and slow the progression of the disease. Treatment options can include blood transfusions, medications, and bone marrow transplant. The best course of treatment will depend on the individual case and the patient's overall health.

It's important for anyone experiencing symptoms of MDS to speak with their healthcare provider, as early diagnosis and treatment can help improve the outlook for the disease. Regular checkups and monitoring can also help catch any changes in the disease early on.

M

yeloproliferative

D

isorders.

Myeloproliferative disorders are a group of blood cancers that affect the production of blood cells in the bone marrow. These disorders cause the bone marrow to produce too many of one or more types of blood cells. This can result in the overproduction of red blood cells, white blood cells, or platelets.

There are several types of myeloproliferative disorders, including:

Polycythemia vera (PV) - PV is a condition in which the bone marrow produces too many red blood cells. This can cause the blood to become thick and increase the risk of blood clots.

Essential thrombocythemia (ET) - ET is a condition in which the bone marrow produces too many platelets. This can cause the blood to thicken and increase the risk of blood clots.

Myelofibrosis (MF) - MF is a condition in which the bone marrow is replaced by scar tissue, which can lead to a decrease in the production of blood cells.

Myeloproliferative disorders are caused by genetic mutations that affect the way blood cells are produced in the bone marrow. The symptoms of these disorders can vary depending on the specific type and the severity of the disease. Some common symptoms of myeloproliferative disorders include fatigue, weakness, dizziness, headache, and shortness of breath.

Treatment for myeloproliferative disorders depends on the type and severity of the disease. Some treatments may include medications to reduce the production of blood cells, chemotherapy, or radiation therapy. In severe cases, a bone marrow transplant may be necessary. Regular check-ups with a doctor and monitoring of blood counts are important for people with myeloproliferative disorders to help manage symptoms and monitor the progression of the disease.

Chapter Three

Who's at risk for Leukemia?

Leukemia can affect anyone, but some factors can increase a person's risk of developing the disease.

One of the most significant risk factors for Leukemia is exposure to radiation, including radiation therapy for cancer treatment, exposure to nuclear fallout, and radiation accidents.

Another risk factor is exposure to certain chemicals, such as benzene, which is commonly found in gasoline, pesticides, and other chemicals used in manufacturing.

Genetic factors can also play a role in Leukemia development, with certain genetic abnormalities and inherited conditions increasing the risk. For example, Down syndrome is associated with a higher risk of developing Leukemia.

Other risk factors include smoking, family history of the disease, and some viruses, such as the human T-cell Leukemia virus (HTLV-1).

It is important to note that having one or more risk factors does not necessarily mean a person will develop Leukemia, and many cases of Leukemia occur in people without any known risk factors.

How do you get

be prevented?

There is no known way to prevent Leukemia. However, there are certain risk factors that can increase the likelihood of developing the disease, and some steps can be taken to reduce exposure to these risk factors.

One risk factor is exposure to certain chemicals and substances, such as benzene and formaldehyde, which are commonly found in workplaces. Individuals who work in industries such as manufacturing, oil refining, and rubber production are at an increased risk of exposure to these chemicals. Taking steps to minimize exposure to these substances, such as wearing protective clothing and following safety guidelines, can help reduce the risk of Leukemia.

Radiation exposure is another risk factor for Leukemia. This can be due to previous cancer treatments, such as radiation therapy or chemotherapy, or exposure to high levels of radiation in the environment, such as living near a nuclear power plant. Reducing exposure to radiation by avoiding unnecessary medical tests that involve radiation and living in areas with low levels of radiation can help lower the risk of Leukemia.

Certain genetic factors can also increase the risk of developing Leukemia. While genetic predisposition to Leukemia cannot be prevented, individuals with a family history of the disease should speak with their healthcare provider about ways to monitor and manage their risk.

Maintaining a healthy lifestyle can also help reduce the risk of developing Leukemia. This includes eating a balanced diet, getting regular exercise, and avoiding smoking and excessive alcohol consumption. Regular check-ups with a healthcare provider can help catch Leukemia early and provide the best chance for successful treatment.

How is

Leukemia

diagnosed?

Leukemia is diagnosed through a series of tests that involve physical examination, blood tests, bone marrow biopsy, and imaging tests. During a physical exam, a doctor will check for signs of an enlarged liver or spleen, swollen lymph nodes, or any other physical abnormalities. Blood tests can detect abnormal blood cells or low blood counts, which can be a sign of Leukemia.

If Leukemia is suspected, a bone marrow biopsy may be necessary to confirm the diagnosis. During a bone marrow biopsy, a small sample of bone marrow and bone is removed with a needle and examined under a microscope. This can help identify any abnormal cells or chromosomal abnormalities that may be indicative of Leukemia.

Imaging tests, such as X-rays, CT scans, or MRI scans, may also be used to detect abnormalities in the body that could be caused by Leukemia. Once a diagnosis has been made, doctors will work with the patient to develop a treatment plan tailored to their specific type and stage of Leukemia.

Medical History and Physical Examination

Medical history and physical examination are important components in the diagnosis of leukemia. Medical history includes gathering information about the patient's past medical conditions, family history, and lifestyle factors that may increase the risk of leukemia. Physical examination involves a thorough examination of the body to look for signs and symptoms of leukemia.

Medical History:

During the medical history, the doctor may ask questions about the patient's past medical conditions, including any history of cancer, chemotherapy, or radiation therapy. The doctor may also inquire about any family history of leukemia or other cancers.

The doctor may ask about lifestyle factors that may increase the risk of leukemia, such as exposure to chemicals or radiation, smoking, and certain medical conditions such as Down syndrome. The doctor may also inquire about the patient's symptoms, such as fatigue, fever, and unexplained weight loss.

Physical Examination:

Physical examination involves a thorough examination of the body to look for signs and symptoms of leukemia. The doctor will examine the skin, lymph nodes, and organs such as the spleen and liver.

The doctor may look for signs of anemia, such as pale skin and fatigue, and signs of bleeding or bruising, such as petechiae and ecchymoses. The doctor may also look for signs of infection, such as fever and enlarged lymph nodes.

The doctor may palpate the abdomen to check for any organ enlargement or tenderness. The doctor may also check for signs of neurological complications, such as headaches and confusion.

Laboratory Tests:

In addition to medical history and physical examination, laboratory tests are important in the diagnosis of leukemia. Blood tests can help determine the number and type of blood cells in the body, and can also detect abnormalities in blood cells.

Bone marrow biopsy involves the removal of a small sample of bone marrow from the hipbone or breastbone. This sample is then examined under a microscope to determine the number and type of blood cells in the bone marrow. A bone marrow biopsy can help diagnose leukemia and determine the stage of the disease.

Imaging Studies:

Imaging studies such as X-rays, CT scans, and MRIs can help doctors detect abnormalities in the body, such as enlarged lymph nodes and organs. These abnormalities can be indicative of leukemia.

medical history and physical examination are important components in the diagnosis of leukemia. During the medical history, the doctor may ask questions about the patient's past medical conditions, family history, and lifestyle factors that may increase the risk of leukemia. Physical examination involves a thorough examination of the body to look for signs and symptoms of leukemia. Laboratory tests and imaging studies can also help diagnose leukemia and determine the stage of the disease. Early diagnosis of leukemia is important in improving the chances of a successful outcome.

Laboratory Tests

Laboratory tests play a crucial role in the diagnosis and monitoring of leukemia. Leukemia is a type of cancer that affects the blood-forming cells in the bone marrow. Laboratory tests can help doctors determine the type and stage of leukemia, monitor the response to treatment, and detect any potential complications. Here are some of the common laboratory tests used in the diagnosis and management of leukemia:

Complete Blood Count (CBC):

A complete blood count (CBC) is a blood test that measures the number and type of blood cells in the body. A CBC can help determine if a person has leukemia by identifying abnormalities in the blood cells. For example, people with leukemia may have an increased number of abnormal white blood cells, a decreased number of red blood cells, and a decreased number of platelets.

Blood Smear:

A blood smear is a laboratory test that involves placing a small drop of blood on a microscope slide and examining it under a microscope. This test can help identify the type of leukemia by looking at the shape and size of the blood cells.

Bone Marrow Biopsy:

A bone marrow biopsy involves the removal of a small sample of bone marrow from the hipbone or breastbone. This sample is then examined under a microscope to determine the number and type of blood cells in the bone marrow. A bone marrow biopsy can help diagnose leukemia and determine the stage of the disease.

Flow Cytometry:

Flow cytometry is a laboratory test that can help identify the number and type of cells in a blood or bone marrow sample. This test can help diagnose leukemia and determine the type and stage of the disease.

Cytogenetic Analysis:

Cytogenetic analysis involves the examination of chromosomes in blood or bone marrow cells. This test can help identify abnormalities in chromosomes, which can be indicative of leukemia.

Molecular Testing:

Molecular testing involves the examination of DNA and RNA in blood or bone marrow cells. This test can help identify genetic mutations, which can be indicative of leukemia.

Lactate Dehydrogenase (LDH):

Lactate dehydrogenase (LDH) is an enzyme that is found in many tissues in the body, including the blood cells. People with leukemia may have increased levels of LDH in their blood, which can be indicative of the disease.

Coagulation Tests:

Coagulation tests, such as prothrombin time (PT) and activated partial thromboplastin time (aPTT), can help determine if a person with leukemia has an increased risk of bleeding or clotting.

Serum Chemistry Tests:

Serum chemistry tests can help assess the function of organs such as the liver and kidneys, which can be affected by leukemia or its treatment.

laboratory tests play a crucial role in the diagnosis and management of leukemia. Complete blood count, blood smear, bone marrow biopsy, flow cytometry, cytogenetic analysis, molecular testing, LDH, coagulation tests, and serum chemistry tests are some of the common laboratory tests used in the diagnosis and monitoring of leukemia. These tests can help determine the type and stage of leukemia, monitor the response to treatment, and detect any potential complications. Early diagnosis and appropriate monitoring can help improve the chances of a successful outcome for people with leukemia.

Imaging Studies

Imaging studies are an essential part of the diagnostic workup for leukemia. Imaging studies are used to detect the presence of leukemia, determine the extent of the disease, and monitor the response to treatment. Here are some of the common imaging studies used in the diagnosis and management of leukemia:

X-rays:

X-rays use radiation to create images of bones and other tissues. X-rays can help detect bone abnormalities, such as fractures or tumors. In people with leukemia, X-rays can help detect bone abnormalities that are caused by the disease or its treatment.

Computed Tomography (CT) Scans:

CT scans use X-rays and computer technology to create detailed images of the body. CT scans can help detect abnormalities in the organs, lymph nodes, and other tissues. CT scans can also help determine the extent of the disease and monitor the response to treatment.

Magnetic Resonance Imaging (MRI):

MRI uses a powerful magnet and radio waves to create detailed images of the body. MRI can help detect abnormalities in the organs, lymph nodes, and other tissues. MRI can also help determine the extent of the disease and monitor the response to treatment.

Positron Emission Tomography (PET) Scans:

PET scans use a small amount of radioactive material to create images of the body. PET scans can help detect areas of the body that are affected by cancer. PET scans can also help determine the extent of the disease and monitor the response to treatment.

Ultrasound:

Ultrasound uses high-frequency sound waves to create images of the body. Ultrasound can help detect abnormalities in the organs, lymph nodes, and other tissues. Ultrasound can also help guide biopsy procedures.

Bone Scans:

Bone scans use a small amount of radioactive material to create images of the bones. Bone scans can help detect areas of the bones that are affected by cancer. Bone scans can also help determine the extent of the disease and monitor the response to treatment.

Angiography:

Angiography is a type of X-ray that is used to examine the blood vessels in the body. Angiography can help detect abnormalities in the blood vessels, such as blockages or narrowing. Angiography can also help guide treatment procedures, such as chemotherapy.

imaging studies are an essential part of the diagnostic workup for leukemia. X-rays, CT scans, MRI, PET scans, ultrasound, bone scans, and angiography are some of the common imaging studies used in the diagnosis and management of leukemia. These imaging studies can help detect the presence of leukemia, determine the extent of the disease, and monitor the response to treatment. Early diagnosis and appropriate monitoring can help improve the chances of a successful outcome for people with leukemia.

Biopsy and Cytogenetics

Biopsy and cytogenetics are essential diagnostic tools in the management of leukemia. A biopsy is a medical procedure that involves the removal of a small sample of tissue for examination under a microscope. Cytogenetics involves the study of chromosomes in cells to identify genetic abnormalities. These two techniques can help diagnose leukemia, determine the type and stage of the disease, and guide treatment decisions.

Bone Marrow Biopsy:

A bone marrow biopsy is the most common type of biopsy used in the diagnosis of leukemia. In a bone marrow biopsy, a small sample of bone marrow is removed from the hipbone or breastbone using a needle. The sample is then examined under a microscope to determine the number and type of blood cells in the bone marrow. A bone marrow biopsy can help diagnose leukemia and determine the stage of the disease.

Lymph Node Biopsy:

In some cases, a lymph node biopsy may be needed to diagnose leukemia. A lymph node biopsy involves the removal of a small sample of lymph node tissue for examination under a microscope. This procedure is usually performed under local anesthesia.

Cytogenetics:

Cytogenetics is a laboratory technique that involves the study of chromosomes in cells. Chromosomes are the structures in cells that carry genetic information. Cytogenetics can help identify genetic abnormalities that are associated with leukemia. For example, some types of leukemia are associated with a specific chromosomal abnormality, such as the Philadelphia chromosome in chronic myeloid leukemia.

Fluorescence In Situ Hybridization (FISH):

Fluorescence in situ hybridization (FISH) is a laboratory technique that can help identify specific chromosomal abnormalities in cells. FISH uses fluorescent probes that bind to specific chromosomal regions, allowing for the visualization of abnormal chromosomes.

Polymerase Chain Reaction (PCR):

Polymerase chain reaction (PCR) is a laboratory technique that can help identify genetic mutations in cells. PCR can be used to detect specific genetic mutations that are associated with leukemia.

biopsy and cytogenetics are essential diagnostic tools in the management of leukemia. Bone marrow biopsy and lymph node biopsy can help diagnose leukemia and determine the stage of the disease. Cytogenetics can help identify genetic abnormalities that are associated with leukemia, such as chromosomal abnormalities and specific genetic mutations. Fluorescence in situ hybridization (FISH) and polymerase chain reaction (PCR) are laboratory techniques that can help identify specific chromosomal abnormalities and genetic mutations, respectively. These diagnostic tools can help guide treatment decisions and improve the chances of a successful outcome for people with leukemia.

Classification and Staging

Classification and staging are crucial aspects of the diagnosis and management of leukemia. Classification refers to the process of categorizing leukemia based on its type and subtype, while staging refers to the process of determining the extent and severity of the disease. Both classification and staging are essential for selecting the most appropriate treatment options and predicting outcomes.

Classification of Leukemia:

Leukemia can be classified based on the type of white blood cell that is affected and the rate at which the disease progresses. The two main types of white blood cells are lymphocytes and myeloid cells. Leukemia that affects lymphocytes is called lymphocytic leukemia, while leukemia that affects myeloid cells is called myeloid leukemia. Leukemia can also be classified based on the rate at which the disease progresses. Acute leukemia is a rapidly progressing form of leukemia, while chronic leukemia is a slower progressing form of leukemia.

There are four main types of leukemia:

Acute Lymphoblastic Leukemia (ALL):

ALL is a rapidly progressing form of leukemia that affects lymphocytes. It is the most common type of leukemia in children, but it can also occur in adults. The treatment for ALL typically involves chemotherapy and may include radiation therapy and stem cell transplant.

Acute Myeloid Leukemia (AML):

AML is a rapidly progressing form of leukemia that affects myeloid cells. It is more common in adults than in children. The treatment for AML typically involves chemotherapy and may include stem cell transplant.

Chronic Lymphocytic Leukemia (CLL):

CLL is a slowly progressing form of leukemia that affects lymphocytes. It is more common in adults and is typically diagnosed in people over the age of 60. The treatment for CLL depends on the stage of the disease and may include chemotherapy, immunotherapy, and targeted therapy.

Chronic Myeloid Leukemia (CML):

CML is a slowly progressing form of leukemia that affects myeloid cells. It is more common in adults and is typically diagnosed in people over the age of 50. The treatment for CML typically involves targeted therapy, such as tyrosine kinase inhibitors.

Staging of Leukemia:

Staging of leukemia is based on the extent and severity of the disease. The staging process involves the use of various tests and procedures, including imaging studies, laboratory tests, and bone marrow biopsy.

The most commonly used system for staging leukemia is the TNM system, which stands for Tumor, Node, and Metastasis. The TNM system is used to stage solid tumors, but it can also be used to stage leukemia.

The stages of leukemia are as follows:

1. Stage 0: This stage is also called the "pre-leukemia" stage, and there are no visible symptoms. This stage is detected only through blood tests or bone marrow biopsy.

2. Stage I: In this stage, the leukemia cells are present in the blood, but not in the bone marrow. There are usually no visible symptoms.

3. Stage II: In this stage, the leukemia cells are present in both the blood and the bone marrow. There may be mild symptoms, such as fatigue, weakness, or weight loss.

4. Stage III: In this stage, the number of leukemia cells is high in both the blood and bone marrow. There may be moderate to severe symptoms, such as anemia, infections, or bleeding.

5. Stage IV: In this stage, the number of leukemia cells is very high in both the blood and bone marrow. There may be severe symptoms, such as bleeding, infections, or organ failure.

World Health Organization Classification

The World Health Organization (WHO) classification is a widely accepted system for classifying leukemia. The WHO classification system was developed in 2001 and has been updated several times since then. The system categorizes leukemia based on the type of white blood cell that is affected, the rate at which the disease progresses, and the presence or absence of genetic abnormalities.

1. The WHO classification system divides leukemia into two main categories: acute leukemia and chronic leukemia. Acute leukemia is a rapidly progressing form of leukemia, while chronic leukemia is a slower progressing form of leukemia.

Acute Leukemia:

2. Acute leukemia is further classified into two subtypes: acute lymphoblastic leukemia (ALL) and acute myeloid leukemia (AML).

ALL is a type of leukemia that affects lymphocytes, which are a type of white blood cell. It is more common in children than in adults, but it can occur at any age. The WHO classification system categorizes ALL into different subtypes based on the presence or absence of certain genetic abnormalities.

AML is a type of leukemia that affects myeloid cells, which are a type of white blood cell. It is more common in adults than in children. The WHO classification system categorizes AML into different subtypes based on the presence or absence of certain genetic abnormalities.

Chronic Leukemia:

3. Chronic leukemia is further classified into two subtypes: chronic lymphocytic leukemia (CLL) and chronic myeloid leukemia (CML).

CLL is a type of leukemia that affects lymphocytes. It is more common in adults and is typically diagnosed in people over the age of 60. The WHO classification system categorizes CLL into different subtypes based on the presence or absence of certain genetic abnormalities.

CML is a type of leukemia that affects myeloid cells. It is more common in adults and is typically diagnosed in people over the age of 50. The WHO classification system categorizes CML into different phases based on the extent and severity of the disease.

In addition to the main categories, the WHO classification system also includes several other subtypes of leukemia, such as:

4. Myelodysplastic syndromes (MDS): a group of disorders in which the bone marrow does not produce enough healthy blood cells.

5. Myeloproliferative neoplasms (MPN): a group of disorders in which the bone marrow produces too many white blood cells, red blood cells, or platelets.

6. Histiocytic and dendritic cell neoplasms: a group of rare disorders that affect certain types of immune cells.

The WHO classification system also includes a category for unclassifiable leukemias, which are cases that cannot be classified into a specific subtype.

the WHO classification system is a widely accepted system for classifying leukemia. It categorizes leukemia based on the type of white blood cell that is affected, the rate at which the disease progresses, and the presence or absence of genetic abnormalities. The system is helpful in guiding treatment decisions and predicting outcomes for people with leukemia.

Prognostic Factors

Prognostic factors are characteristics of leukemia that are associated with the likelihood of achieving remission and survival. Prognostic factors can help doctors determine the most appropriate treatment plan and predict the outcome of the disease. Several factors contribute to the prognosis of leukemia, including age, sex, overall health, genetic abnormalities, and response to treatment.

Age:

Age is a significant prognostic factor for leukemia. Children and young adults with leukemia generally have a better prognosis than older adults. Older adults are more likely to have other health conditions that can complicate treatment and affect their overall prognosis.

Sex:

Sex is also a prognostic factor for leukemia. Women with leukemia generally have a better prognosis than men. The reason for this difference is not fully understood, but it may be related to hormonal factors or differences in immune function.

Overall Health:

The overall health of a person with leukemia is a significant prognostic factor. People who have other health conditions, such as heart disease or diabetes, may have a more challenging time tolerating chemotherapy and other treatments. Additionally, people who have a weakened immune system may be more susceptible to infections during treatment, which can affect their prognosis.

Genetic Abnormalities:

Genetic abnormalities play a critical role in the prognosis of leukemia. Some genetic abnormalities are associated with a better prognosis, while others are associated with a worse prognosis. For example, people with certain genetic abnormalities, such as the Philadelphia chromosome, have a higher risk of developing leukemia and a poorer prognosis.

Response to Treatment:

Response to treatment is one of the most critical prognostic factors for leukemia. People who respond well to treatment and achieve remission have a better prognosis than those who do not respond well to treatment. The response to treatment is typically evaluated using various tests, such as bone marrow biopsy and imaging studies.

Other factors that may contribute to the prognosis of leukemia include the type and stage of the disease, the presence or absence of specific symptoms, and the treatment approach. For example, people with acute lymphoblastic leukemia (ALL) who have specific genetic abnormalities, such as the t(9;22) or t(4;11) translocations, may have a worse prognosis than those without these abnormalities.

prognostic factors are essential for determining the most appropriate treatment plan and predicting the outcome of leukemia. Age, sex, overall health, genetic abnormalities, and response to treatment are some of the critical prognostic factors that doctors consider when managing leukemia. Understanding these factors can help people with leukemia make informed decisions about their treatment options and prepare for their prognosis.

Staging Systems

Staging systems are used to classify the extent and severity of cancer, including leukemia. Staging helps doctors determine the best course of treatment and provides information on the prognosis of the disease. The staging of leukemia is based on several factors, including the number of abnormal cells in the bone marrow and blood, the presence of symptoms, and the extent of the disease in other parts of the body.

The two primary staging systems used for leukemia are the French-American-British (FAB) classification and the World Health Organization (WHO) classification.

French-American-British (FAB) Classification:

The FAB classification system was developed in the 1970s and is based on the type of white blood cell affected by leukemia. The FAB system divides leukemia into four categories:

Acute lymphoblastic leukemia (ALL)

Acute myeloid leukemia (AML)

Chronic lymphocytic leukemia (CLL)

Chronic myeloid leukemia (CML)

Each category is further divided into subtypes based on the specific cell type and other characteristics.

World Health Organization (WHO) Classification:

1. The WHO classification system was developed in 2001 and updated in 2016. This system categorizes leukemia based on the type of white blood cell affected, the rate at which the disease progresses, and the presence or absence of genetic abnormalities. The WHO system divides leukemia into two main categories: acute leukemia and chronic leukemia.

2. Acute leukemia is further classified into two subtypes: acute lymphoblastic leukemia (ALL) and acute myeloid leukemia (AML). Chron-

ic leukemia is further classified into two subtypes: chronic lymphocytic leukemia (CLL) and chronic myeloid leukemia (CML).

In addition to these main categories, the WHO classification system includes several other subtypes of leukemia, such as myelodysplastic syndromes (MDS) and myeloproliferative neoplasms (MPN).

Stages of Leukemia:

The staging of leukemia is based on several factors, including the number of abnormal cells in the bone marrow and blood, the presence of symptoms, and the extent of the disease in other parts of the body. The stages of leukemia are:

3. Stage 0: The leukemia cells are present in the bone marrow, but there are no symptoms, and the number of abnormal cells is low.

4. Stage I: The leukemia cells are present in the bone marrow, and the number of abnormal cells is moderate.

5. Stage II: The leukemia cells are present in the bone marrow, and the number of abnormal cells is high.

6. Stage III: The leukemia cells are present in the bone marrow, and the number of abnormal cells is very high. The leukemia cells may also be present in the blood and lymph nodes.

7. Stage IV: The leukemia cells have spread to other parts of the body, such as the liver, spleen, and brain.

Treatment of Leukemia:

The treatment of leukemia depends on the type and stage of the disease. Treatment options include chemotherapy, radiation therapy, targeted therapy, stem cell transplantation, and immunotherapy. The goal of treatment is to destroy the leukemia cells and achieve remission.

Prognosis of Leukemia:

The prognosis of leukemia depends on several factors, including the type and stage of the disease, the age and overall health of the person, and the response to treatment. In general, the prognosis is better for people with chronic leukemia than for those with acute leukemia. Additionally, younger people with leukemia tend to have a better prognosis than older adults.

the staging of leukemia is an essential part of determining the most appropriate treatment plan and predicting the outcome of the disease. The FAB and WHO classification systems are the two primary staging systems used.

Chapter Six

How do you treat Leukemia?

Leukemia treatment options depend on several factors, including the type of Leukemia, the extent of the disease, and the individual's overall health. Here are some common treatments for Leukemia:

1. Chemotherapy: Chemotherapy is a common treatment for Leukemia. It involves the use of drugs to kill cancer cells. Chemotherapy is often given in cycles, with periods of rest in between to allow the body to recover.

2. Radiation therapy: Radiation therapy uses high-energy X-rays or other types of radiation to kill cancer cells. It may be used alone or in combination with chemotherapy.

3. Stem cell transplant: A stem cell transplant involves replacing the diseased bone marrow with healthy stem cells. This can be done using stem cells from a donor or the patient's own stem cells.

4. Targeted therapy: Targeted therapy drugs attack specific proteins or genes that help cancer cells grow. They are usually used in combination with chemotherapy or radiation therapy.

5. Immunotherapy: Immunotherapy is a type of cancer treatment that helps the immune system to fight cancer. It involves the use of drugs that stimulate the immune system to attack cancer cells.

6. Surgery: Surgery may be used in rare cases to remove an enlarged spleen or lymph nodes.

It's important to note that the treatment for Leukemia is complex, and patients often receive a combination of treatments to achieve the best possible outcome. The specific treatment plan will depend on the type and stage of the disease, as well as the individual's overall health.

Goals of Treatment

The goals of treatment for leukemia are to eliminate as many leukemia cells as possible, achieve remission, prevent relapse, and improve quality of life. The specific goals of treatment may vary depending on the type and stage of leukemia, as well as the age and overall health of the patient. In general, the goals of treatment are to improve the patient's chances of survival and minimize the side effects of treatment.

Eliminating Leukemia Cells:

The primary goal of leukemia treatment is to eliminate as many leukemia cells as possible from the body. This can be achieved through a variety of treatment options, including chemotherapy, radiation therapy, targeted therapy, stem cell transplantation, and immunotherapy. The goal is to destroy the leukemia cells and prevent them from growing and spreading.

Achieving Remission:

Remission is a state in which there is no evidence of leukemia in the body. The goal of treatment is to achieve remission as quickly as possible. This can be achieved through a variety of treatment options, including chemotherapy, radiation therapy, targeted therapy, stem cell transplantation, and immunotherapy. Once remission is achieved, patients will need to continue treatment to prevent relapse.

Preventing Relapse:

The risk of relapse varies depending on the type and stage of leukemia. The goal of treatment is to prevent relapse by continuing treatment after remission is achieved. This can include maintenance chemotherapy, stem cell transplantation, or immunotherapy. Close monitoring of the patient's health and regular follow-up appointments are also important for preventing relapse.

Improving Quality of Life:

Leukemia and its treatments can cause a variety of side effects that can affect a patient's quality of life. The goal of treatment is to minimize the side effects of treatment and improve the patient's quality of life. This can include managing symptoms such as nausea, fatigue, and pain, as well as providing emotional and psychological support.

Overall Survival:

The ultimate goal of leukemia treatment is to improve overall survival. Survival rates vary depending on the type and stage of leukemia, as well as the age and overall health of the patient. In general, the earlier the leukemia is diagnosed and treated, the better the chances of survival.

In addition to the goals of treatment, it is important for patients to be actively involved in their own care. This includes maintaining a healthy lifestyle, following the treatment plan prescribed by their healthcare provider, and reporting any new or unusual symptoms. Patients should also communicate openly with their healthcare team and ask questions about their treatment options and the goals of treatment.

the goals of treatment for leukemia are to eliminate as many leukemia cells as possible, achieve remission, prevent relapse, and improve quality of life. The specific goals of treatment may vary depending on the type and stage of leukemia, as well as the age and overall health of the patient. The ultimate goal is to improve overall survival and provide the best possible care for patients with leukemia.

Multidisciplinary Approach

Leukemia is a complex disease that requires a multidisciplinary approach for effective treatment. A multidisciplinary approach involves a team of healthcare professionals from various specialties working together to provide comprehensive care for patients with leukemia. The team may include hematologists, oncologists, radiologists, pathologists, nurses, social workers, and other healthcare professionals, depending on the specific needs of the patient.

The multidisciplinary approach to leukemia treatment is important for several reasons. First, leukemia is a complex disease that requires a comprehensive understanding of the disease and its treatment options. By bringing together healthcare professionals from different specialties, patients can receive a more holistic approach to their care that takes into account all aspects of their disease and their overall health.

Second, leukemia treatment often involves a combination of different treatment options, such as chemotherapy, radiation therapy, targeted therapy, stem cell transplantation, and immunotherapy. These treatments can have significant side effects and require close monitoring and management. A multidisciplinary team can work together to provide the best possible care for patients and minimize the side effects of treatment.

Third, leukemia can have significant psychological and social impacts on patients and their families. A multidisciplinary team can provide emotional and psychological support, as well as social services, to help patients and their families cope with the challenges of leukemia treatment.

Finally, a multidisciplinary approach can improve communication and coordination among healthcare professionals, leading to more effective and efficient care for patients. This can lead to better outcomes and improved quality of life for patients with leukemia.

The specific roles of healthcare professionals in a multidisciplinary team may vary depending on the type and stage of leukemia, as well as the needs of the patient. However, some of the key roles of healthcare professionals in a multidisciplinary team for leukemia treatment include:

Hematologists/Oncologists:

Hematologists and oncologists are medical doctors who specialize in the diagnosis and treatment of blood cancers, including leukemia. They are responsible for overseeing the patient's treatment plan and coordinating care with other healthcare professionals. They may also perform bone marrow biopsies and other diagnostic tests to monitor the patient's disease.

Radiologists:

Radiologists specialize in the use of imaging technologies, such as CT scans, MRIs, and PET scans, to diagnose and monitor diseases. They may perform imaging tests to help diagnose leukemia and monitor the patient's response to treatment.

Pathologists:

Pathologists specialize in the study of tissues and cells to diagnose diseases. They may analyze bone marrow samples and other tissue samples to confirm the diagnosis of leukemia and monitor the patient's disease.

Nurses:

Nurses play a critical role in the care of patients with leukemia. They may administer chemotherapy and other treatments, monitor the patient's vital signs, and manage the patient's side effects of treatment. They also provide emotional support and education to patients and their families.

Social Workers:

Social workers provide emotional and practical support to patients and their families. They may assist with financial and insurance issues, help patients navigate the healthcare system, and provide counseling and other support services.

a multidisciplinary approach is essential for the effective treatment of leukemia. A team of healthcare professionals from various specialties can provide comprehensive care that takes into account all aspects of the disease and the patient's overall health. By working together, healthcare professionals can provide the best possible care for patients with leukemia and improve their quality of life.

Factors Influencing Treatment Decisions

Leukemia treatment decisions are complex and can be influenced by a variety of factors, including the type and stage of the disease, the patient's age and overall health, the potential benefits and risks of treatment, and the patient's personal preferences and values. In this essay, we will explore some of the factors that can influence leukemia treatment decisions.

Type and Stage of Leukemia

The type and stage of leukemia can have a significant impact on treatment decisions. Acute leukemias, such as acute lymphoblastic leukemia (ALL) and acute myeloid leukemia (AML), require immediate treatment because they progress rapidly and can be life-threatening. Chronic leukemias, such as chronic lymphocytic leukemia (CLL) and chronic myeloid leukemia

(CML), may not require immediate treatment, and the decision to treat is based on the stage of the disease and the patient's overall health.

The treatment options for leukemia vary depending on the type of leukemia. Chemotherapy is the standard treatment for most types of leukemia, but some patients may benefit from other treatments, such as radiation therapy, targeted therapy, stem cell transplantation, or immunotherapy. The decision to use a particular treatment or combination of treatments depends on the type and stage of the leukemia, as well as the potential benefits and risks of each treatment.

Age and Overall Health

The patient's age and overall health are important factors in leukemia treatment decisions. Older patients and patients with other health conditions may not be able to tolerate certain treatments or may be at a higher risk of complications from treatment. In these cases, the treatment plan may need to be modified or alternative treatments may be considered.

Younger patients may be able to tolerate more aggressive treatments, such as high-dose chemotherapy or stem cell transplantation, which may offer the best chance of a cure. However, these treatments can have significant side effects and long-term complications, so the decision to use them must be carefully considered in light of the potential benefits and risks.

Potential Benefits and Risks of Treatment

The potential benefits and risks of leukemia treatment are important factors in treatment decisions. Chemotherapy and other treatments can have significant side effects, such as nausea, vomiting, hair loss, and increased risk of infection. Some treatments can also have long-term effects, such as infertility, heart damage, or secondary cancers.

The potential benefits of treatment, such as improved survival or quality of life, must be weighed against the potential risks and side effects. The decision to treat may also depend on the patient's goals and priorities, such as whether the patient is seeking a cure or simply wants to manage symptoms and prolong life.

Personal Preferences and Values

Personal preferences and values can also influence leukemia treatment decisions. Some patients may prefer to avoid aggressive treatments that have significant side effects, while others may want to do everything possible to achieve a cure. Patients may also have cultural or religious beliefs that influence their treatment decisions.

Shared decision-making, in which the patient and healthcare team work together to make treatment decisions, is becoming increasingly common in leukemia treatment. This approach takes into account the patient's personal preferences and values, as well as the medical evidence and expertise of the healthcare team.

leukemia treatment decisions are complex and can be influenced by a variety of factors, including the type and stage of the disease, the patient's age and overall health, the potential benefits and risks of treatment, and the patient's personal preferences and values. A multidisciplinary team of healthcare professionals can help patients navigate these factors and make informed decisions about their treatment. Shared decision-making can ensure that the patient's values and preferences are taken into account, leading to more personalized and effective care.

Chemotherapy for

Leukemia

patients

Chemotherapy is one of the primary treatments for Leukemia, as it uses powerful drugs to kill cancer cells in the body. The drugs are usually given intravenously, but they can also be taken in pill form. Chemotherapy can be given alone or in combination with other treatments such as radiation therapy, stem cell transplants, or targeted therapy.

The goal of chemotherapy is to destroy as many cancer cells as possible while minimizing the damage to healthy cells. The treatment is usually given in cycles of several days, followed by a period of rest to allow the body to recover. The number of cycles and the duration of treatment depend on the type and stage of Leukemia.

Chemotherapy drugs can cause side effects, as they can damage normal cells along with cancer cells. The most common side effects are hair loss, fatigue, nausea, vomiting, and loss of appetite. Other side effects may include mouth sores, infection, bleeding, and an increased risk of developing other cancers.

To manage the side effects of chemotherapy, patients may be given medications to relieve symptoms and support their immune system. They may also need blood transfusions or platelet transfusions to replace the blood cells that are destroyed by the chemotherapy.

It is important for patients to work closely with their healthcare team to manage the side effects of chemotherapy and ensure that they receive the best possible care. Chemotherapy can be an effective treatment for Leukemia, but it requires careful monitoring and management to minimize its impact on the patient's overall health and well-being.

Radiation therapy for

Leukemia

patients

Radiation therapy is another treatment option for Leukemia patients, especially those with Leukemia in specific areas of the body. In this treatment, high-energy radiation is used to kill Leukemia cells and shrink tumors.

External beam radiation therapy is the most common type of radiation therapy used for Leukemia. During this treatment, a machine outside the body delivers radiation to the affected area. The treatment is usually done in several sessions over a period of weeks.

Radiation therapy may be used alone or in combination with other treatments, such as chemotherapy or stem cell transplant. It may also be used to prepare patients for a stem cell transplant by destroying Leukemia cells in the bone marrow.

As with chemotherapy, radiation therapy can cause side effects, including fatigue, skin irritation, and damage to healthy cells in the treated area. The specific side effects will depend on the location and amount of radiation used.

Bone marrow and stem cell transplants for

Leukemia

patients

Bone marrow and stem cell transplants are often used as a treatment option for Leukemia patients. The purpose of a transplant is to replace the patient's diseased or damaged bone marrow with healthy bone marrow from a donor.

During a transplant, the patient will receive high doses of chemotherapy and/or radiation therapy to kill off their diseased bone marrow. Then, they will receive a transplant of healthy bone marrow from a donor. The bone marrow can be collected from the patient themselves (autologous transplant) or from a donor (allogeneic transplant).

In an allogeneic transplant, the donor must have a tissue type that closely matches the patient's. This is to reduce the risk of the patient's immune system attacking the transplanted bone marrow, a process known as graft-versus-host disease (GVHD).

After the transplant, the patient will need to be monitored closely for signs of GVHD and other complications. They will also need to take medications to suppress their immune system, to prevent their body from attacking the transplanted bone marrow.

Bone marrow and stem cell transplants can be a potentially curative treatment option for Leukemia, but they can also come with significant risks and side effects. It is important for patients to discuss the potential risks and benefits with their healthcare team before undergoing a transplant.

Immunotherapy and targeted therapy for

Leukemia

patients

Immunotherapy and targeted therapy are two more recent approaches to treating Leukemia that have shown promising results.

Immunotherapy works by helping the body's own immune system fight the cancer cells. There are several types of immunotherapy for Leukemia, including monoclonal antibodies, which are synthetic versions of immune system proteins that can target specific cancer cells. These antibodies can either kill the cancer cells directly or signal the immune system to attack the cells.

Another type of immunotherapy is chimeric antigen receptor (CAR) T-cell therapy, which involves extracting a patient's own T-cells (a type of immune cell) and genetically modifying them to target specific cancer cells. These modified T-cells are then infused back into the patient's body to help fight the cancer.

Targeted therapy, on the other hand, involves using drugs that specifically target certain proteins or genes that are involved in the growth and survival of cancer cells. By targeting these specific factors, targeted therapy can help stop the growth and spread of Leukemia cells while minimizing damage to healthy cells.

Both immunotherapy and targeted therapy have shown promising results in the treatment of Leukemia, particularly in cases where other treatments have not been successful. However, like other forms of treatment, they can come with side effects and may not be suitable for every patient. A healthcare provider will evaluate the patient's individual situation and determine the most appropriate treatment plan.

Induction Therapy

Induction therapy is the initial phase of treatment for acute leukemias, such as acute lymphoblastic leukemia (ALL) and acute myeloid leukemia (AML). The goal of induction therapy is to achieve remission, which means that there is no evidence of leukemia cells in the bone marrow and blood. In this essay, we will explore how induction therapy works, the drugs used in induction therapy, and the potential side effects and complications of induction therapy.

How Induction Therapy Works

Induction therapy for acute leukemias typically involves a combination of chemotherapy drugs, given over several weeks. The drugs used in induction therapy are designed to kill leukemia cells and reduce the number of leukemia cells in the bone marrow and blood. Once remission is achieved, patients may undergo consolidation therapy, which is designed to further reduce the number of leukemia cells in the body and prevent relapse.

The drugs used in induction therapy can be given orally, intravenously, or by injection into the spinal fluid. Combination chemotherapy is often used for induction therapy, because it can be more effective than single-agent chemotherapy. The combination of drugs used depends on the type and stage of the leukemia, as well as the patient's overall health and potential side effects.

Drugs Used in Induction Therapy

The drugs commonly used in induction therapy for acute leukemias include:

1. Anthracyclines: These drugs, such as daunorubicin and doxorubicin, work by damaging the DNA of cancer cells, leading to cell death.

2. Cytarabine: This drug works by blocking DNA synthesis in cancer cells, leading to cell death.

3. Thioguanine: This drug works by interfering with DNA synthesis in cancer cells, leading to cell death.

4. Vincristine: This drug works by disrupting the cell division process in cancer cells, leading to cell death.

5. Prednisone: This drug is a type of corticosteroid that can help kill leukemia cells and reduce inflammation.

The combination of drugs used in induction therapy may vary depending on the type and stage of the leukemia, as well as the patient's overall health and potential side effects.

Side Effects and Complications

Induction therapy can have side effects, which can vary depending on the type and dose of chemotherapy drugs used. Common side effects of induction therapy for acute leukemias include:

Nausea and vomiting

Hair loss

Fatigue

Increased risk of infection

Anemia

Easy bruising or bleeding

Mouth sores

Loss of appetite

Induction therapy can also have long-term side effects, such as infertility, heart damage, or secondary cancers. The risk of long-term side effects depends on the type and dose of chemotherapy drugs used, as well as the patient's age and overall health.

Induction therapy can also increase the risk of infection, because it can damage the bone marrow, which produces white blood cells that fight infection. Patients undergoing induction therapy may need to take precautions to avoid infection, such as avoiding crowds and washing their hands frequently.

In rare cases, induction therapy can cause serious complications, such as an allergic reaction, kidney or liver damage, or blood clots. Patients undergoing induction therapy should be closely monitored for these complications and should report any symptoms or side effects to their healthcare team.

induction therapy is the initial phase of treatment for acute leukemias, designed to achieve remission by reducing the number of leukemia cells in the bone marrow and blood. The drugs used in induction therapy can have side effects and complications, which can vary depending on the type and dose of chemotherapy drugs used. Patients undergoing induction therapy should be closely monitored for side effects and complications, and should report any symptoms to their health professional.

Consolidation and Maintenance Therapy

Consolidation and maintenance therapy are two additional phases of treatment for acute leukemias, such as acute lymphoblastic leukemia (ALL) and acute myeloid leukemia (AML). These phases of treatment are designed to further reduce the number of leukemia cells in the body and prevent relapse. In this essay, we will explore how consolidation and maintenance therapy work, the drugs used in these treatments, and the potential side effects and complications.

How Consolidation Therapy Works

Consolidation therapy is the second phase of treatment for acute leukemias, following induction therapy. The goal of consolidation therapy is to further reduce the number of leukemia cells in the body and prevent relapse. This is achieved through the use of high-dose chemotherapy, which can be more effective than the lower doses used in induction therapy.

The drugs used in consolidation therapy may be the same as those used in induction therapy, or they may be different. The choice of drugs depends on the type and stage of the leukemia, as well as the patient's overall health and potential side effects. The drugs may be given orally, intravenously, or by injection into the spinal fluid.

Consolidation therapy can have side effects, which can vary depending on the type and dose of chemotherapy drugs used. Common side effects of consolidation therapy for acute leukemias include:

- Nausea and vomiting
- Fatigue
- Increased risk of infection
- Anemia
- Easy bruising or bleeding
- Mouth sores
- Loss of appetite

Patients undergoing consolidation therapy may also be at risk for long-term side effects, such as infertility, heart damage, or secondary cancers.

How Maintenance Therapy Works

Maintenance therapy is the third phase of treatment for acute leukemias, following induction and consolidation therapy. The goal of maintenance therapy is to prevent relapse by continuing treatment with low-dose chemotherapy drugs for a period of months or years.

The drugs used in maintenance therapy may be the same as those used in induction and consolidation therapy, or they may be different. The choice of drugs depends on the type and stage of the leukemia, as well as the patient's overall health and potential side effects. The drugs may be given orally, intravenously, or by injection into the spinal fluid.

Maintenance therapy can have side effects, which can vary depending on the type and dose of chemotherapy drugs used. Common side effects of maintenance therapy for acute leukemias include:

- Nausea and vomiting
- Fatigue
- Increased risk of infection
- Anemia
- Easy bruising or bleeding
- Mouth sores
- Loss of appetite

Patients undergoing maintenance therapy may also be at risk for long-term side effects, such as infertility, heart damage, or secondary cancers.

Combination Therapy

Combination therapy, which involves the use of multiple chemotherapy drugs, is often used in consolidation and maintenance therapy. This is because combination therapy can be more effective than single-agent chemotherapy.

Combination therapy can also increase the risk of side effects and complications, such as an increased risk of infection or damage to the heart or other organs. Patients undergoing combination therapy should be closely monitored for side effects and complications, and should report any symptoms to their healthcare team.

consolidation and maintenance therapy are two additional phases of treatment for acute leukemias, designed to further reduce the number of leukemia cells in the body and prevent relapse. These phases of treatment involve the use of high-dose and low-dose chemotherapy drugs, respectively, and can have side effects and complications. Patients undergoing consolidation and maintenance therapy should be closely monitored for side effects and complications, and should report any symptoms to their healthcare team.

Targeted Therapy

Targeted therapy is a type of cancer treatment that aims to identify and attack cancer cells specifically, while minimizing damage to healthy cells. This approach differs from traditional chemotherapy, which kills cancer cells along with healthy cells.

In leukemia, targeted therapy can be used to attack the specific molecular or genetic abnormalities that are causing the cancer cells to grow and divide uncontrollably. This approach has shown promising results in some types of leukemia, particularly chronic myeloid leukemia (CML) and acute lymphoblastic leukemia (ALL).

One of the most successful targeted therapies for leukemia is imatinib, which is used to treat CML. Imatinib targets a specific enzyme called BCR-ABL, which is produced by a genetic abnormality known as the Philadelphia chromosome. By inhibiting BCR-ABL, imatinib can prevent the growth and division of cancer cells. Imatinib has revolutionized the treatment of CML, with many patients experiencing long-term remission.

Another targeted therapy used in leukemia is monoclonal antibodies. These drugs are designed to target specific proteins on the surface of cancer cells, which can then be attacked by the immune system. One example is rituximab, which is used to treat some types of non-Hodgkin lymphoma and chronic lymphocytic leukemia. Rituximab targets a protein called CD20, which is found on the surface of B cells, a type of white blood cell that can become cancerous in some types of leukemia.

Another type of targeted therapy is small-molecule inhibitors. These drugs are designed to target specific molecules within cancer cells that are essential for their growth and survival. One example is venetoclax, which is used to treat chronic lymphocytic leukemia. Venetoclax targets a protein called B-cell lymphoma 2 (BCL-2), which helps cancer cells to survive by preventing them from undergoing programmed cell death.

While targeted therapy has shown great promise in the treatment of leukemia, it is important to note that it is not a one-size-fits-all approach. Different types of leukemia have different molecular and genetic abnormalities, and the effectiveness of targeted therapy depends on identifying the specific abnormality driving the cancer cells' growth and division.

In addition, targeted therapy can have side effects, just like traditional chemotherapy. Common side effects include fatigue, nausea, vomiting, and diarrhea. However, because targeted therapy is more selective in its targeting of cancer cells, it may have fewer side effects than traditional chemotherapy.

In summary, targeted therapy is a promising approach to the treatment of leukemia. By identifying and attacking specific molecular and genetic abnormalities within cancer cells, targeted therapy can be more effective and have fewer side effects than traditional chemotherapy. While it is not a one-size-fits-all approach, targeted therapy has shown great promise in the treatment of certain types of leukemia, and it is likely to play an increasingly important role in the management of this disease in the future.

External Beam Radiation

External beam radiation therapy is a type of cancer treatment that uses high-energy X-rays or other types of radiation to kill cancer cells. This type of therapy is commonly used to treat solid tumors, but it can also be used to treat certain types of leukemia.

In external beam radiation therapy, the radiation is delivered to the patient from a machine called a linear accelerator. The machine delivers the radiation in precise doses, over a period of several weeks. The patient lies on a table while the machine moves around them, delivering the radiation to the affected area.

External beam radiation therapy can be used to treat leukemia in a few different ways. For example, it may be used to treat leukemia that has spread to other parts of the body, such as the brain or bones. In these cases, the radiation is delivered to the affected area in order to kill the cancer cells and shrink the tumors.

External beam radiation therapy can also be used to prepare a patient for a stem cell transplant. In this case, the radiation is delivered to the patient's bone marrow in order to kill the cancer cells and make room for the new, healthy stem cells.

External beam radiation therapy can have side effects, depending on the area of the body being treated and the dose of radiation being used. Common side effects include fatigue, skin irritation, and nausea. Patients may also experience long-term effects, such as a higher risk of developing a secondary cancer or damage to nearby organs.

In summary, external beam radiation therapy is a type of cancer treatment that uses high-energy X-rays or other types of radiation to kill cancer cells. It can be used to treat leukemia that has spread to other parts of the body, as well as to prepare a patient for a stem cell transplant. While it can have side effects, external beam radiation therapy is an important tool in the fight against leukemia, and it has helped many patients achieve remission or long-term survival.

Radioimmunotherapy

Radioimmunotherapy is a type of cancer treatment that combines radiation therapy and immunotherapy. This treatment uses a radioactive substance attached to an antibody that targets specific cancer cells. When the antibody binds to the cancer cells, the radioactive substance delivers radiation directly to the tumor cells, killing them.

Radioimmunotherapy has been used to treat a variety of cancers, including leukemia. It is particularly effective in treating leukemia because the radioactive substance can penetrate the bone marrow and target the leukemia cells there.

One example of radioimmunotherapy for leukemia is the drug ibritumomab tiuxetan. This drug is used to treat certain types of non-Hodgkin lymphoma, which is a type of cancer that affects the lymphatic system. The drug works by attaching to a protein called CD20 on the surface of cancer cells. The radioactive substance then delivers radiation directly to the cancer cells, killing them.

Another example is the drug Zevalin, which is also used to treat non-Hodgkin lymphoma. This drug works in a similar way to ibritumomab tiuxetan, by attaching to the CD20 protein on cancer cells and delivering radiation to the cells.

Radioimmunotherapy can have side effects, including fatigue, nausea, and a higher risk of infection. However, because the treatment is targeted specifically to cancer cells, it can cause less damage to healthy tissues than other types of radiation therapy.

Radioimmunotherapy is a promising treatment option for leukemia and other cancers. It is still being studied in clinical trials, and researchers are working to improve its effectiveness and reduce its side effects. In some cases, radioimmunotherapy may be used in combination with other treatments, such as chemotherapy, to improve outcomes for patients.

In summary, radioimmunotherapy is a type of cancer treatment that combines radiation therapy and immunotherapy. It has been used to treat leukemia and other types of cancer by targeting specific cancer cells with a radioactive substance attached to an antibody. While it can have side effects, radioimmunotherapy is a promising treatment option that can be effective in killing cancer cells while causing less damage to healthy tissues.

Total Body Irradiation

Total body irradiation (TBI) is a type of radiation therapy that is used in the treatment of leukemia, lymphoma, and other types of cancer. It involves the use of high-energy radiation to destroy cancer cells throughout the entire body. TBI is often used in conjunction with chemotherapy and stem cell transplantation to achieve remission and improve survival rates.

TBI works by damaging the DNA of cancer cells, which leads to their death. The radiation used in TBI is delivered to the entire body, rather than to a specific area, and is usually given in multiple doses over a period of several days. The goal of TBI is to kill as many cancer cells as possible while minimizing damage to healthy cells.

1. There are two types of TBI: high-dose and low-dose. High-dose TBI is typically given prior to stem cell transplantation and is used to destroy any remaining cancer cells in the body before the transplant. Low-dose TBI is used in conjunction with chemotherapy to treat leukemia and lymphoma that has spread throughout the body.

The procedure for TBI involves the patient lying on a table while a machine delivers the radiation. The patient is usually positioned in such a way as to minimize the amount of radiation exposure to healthy tissues and organs. The treatment itself is painless, but patients may experience side effects such as nausea, fatigue, and skin irritation.

One of the advantages of TBI is its ability to target cancer cells throughout the entire body. This is particularly useful in cases where the cancer has spread to multiple organs or if there is a high risk of the cancer spreading.

TBI can also be used as a conditioning treatment before stem cell transplantation, which can improve the success of the transplant.

However, TBI also has some drawbacks. Because it targets the entire body, it can damage healthy tissues and organs, leading to side effects such as infertility, cataracts, and increased risk of developing other cancers. Patients who undergo TBI may also experience long-term effects such as cognitive impairment and decreased lung function.

In addition, TBI may not be suitable for all patients. Those who are pregnant or who have certain medical conditions, such as heart disease or lung disease, may not be able to tolerate the treatment. Patients who have previously received radiation therapy may also be at increased risk for side effects from TBI.

Overall, TBI is a powerful tool in the treatment of leukemia and other cancers. It can be an effective way to target cancer cells throughout the entire body and improve survival rates. However, it is important for patients to be aware of the potential risks and side effects associated with the treatment, and to work closely with their healthcare team to determine whether TBI is the best option for their specific situation.

Stem Cell Transplantation

Stem cell transplantation is a medical procedure that involves the transfer of healthy stem cells from a donor to a patient with a damaged or diseased bone marrow. This procedure is used in the treatment of several blood-related disorders, including leukemia. In this essay, we will explore the use of stem cell transplantation in the treatment of leukemia.

Leukemia is a cancer of the blood and bone marrow, characterized by the uncontrolled production of abnormal white blood cells. Stem cell transplantation is a treatment option for leukemia patients who have failed to respond to other treatments or who have relapsed after initial treatment. The procedure involves the replacement of the patient's damaged bone marrow with healthy stem cells from a donor. The new stem cells will then develop into healthy blood cells in the patient's body.

1. There are two types of stem cell transplantation: autologous and allogeneic. Autologous stem cell transplantation involves the use of the patient's own stem cells, which are harvested and then reinfused after high-dose chemotherapy. Allogeneic stem cell transplantation, on the other hand, involves the use of stem cells from a donor, which are matched to the patient's tissue type.

Allogeneic stem cell transplantation is the preferred treatment for leukemia, as it has a higher chance of achieving a cure. However, the procedure is associated with a higher risk of complications, including graft-versus-host disease (GVHD), a condition in which the donor's immune cells attack the patient's normal tissues.

Before the transplantation procedure, the patient undergoes several tests to determine the compatibility of the donor's stem cells. The donor is typically a close relative, but in some cases, unrelated donors may be used. The patient is also given high-dose chemotherapy or radiation therapy to destroy any remaining cancer cells and suppress the patient's immune system, allowing the donor's stem cells to take hold and produce new, healthy blood cells.

The transplantation procedure itself involves the infusion of the donor's stem cells through a vein in the patient's arm. The stem cells then travel to the patient's bone marrow and begin to produce new blood cells. The patient may experience side effects, such as nausea, vomiting, and fatigue, as well as an increased risk of infection due to the weakened immune system.

After the transplantation, the patient is monitored closely for any signs of complications or rejection of the donor's stem cells. The patient may also require supportive care, such as blood transfusions, antibiotics, and anti-rejection medications. It can take several weeks or months for the patient's blood counts to recover, and during this time, the patient is at an increased risk of infection.

stem cell transplantation is a valuable treatment option for leukemia patients who have failed to respond to other treatments or who have relapsed after initial treatment. The procedure involves the replacement of the patient's damaged bone marrow with healthy stem cells from a donor. While allogeneic stem cell transplantation has a higher chance of achieving a cure, it is also associated with a higher risk of complications. Therefore, careful patient selection and monitoring are essential for a successful outcome.

Autologous Transplant

Autologous stem cell transplantation is a treatment option for patients with leukemia who have undergone high-dose chemotherapy. Autologous transplantation involves the use of a patient's own stem cells, which are collected prior to the administration of high-dose chemotherapy. The stem cells are then reinfused back into the patient's body following chemotherapy. This approach allows for the recovery of the patient's blood-forming cells that were destroyed during the chemotherapy. Autologous stem cell transplantation offers several advantages over other types of transplantation, such as reduced risk of rejection, infection, and graft-versus-host disease.

Before undergoing autologous transplantation, patients must undergo an extensive evaluation to ensure that they are eligible for the procedure. This evaluation typically includes a physical examination, blood tests, imaging studies, and other tests to assess the patient's overall health and the extent of the leukemia.

The collection of stem cells is typically done through a process called leukapheresis. During this procedure, blood is removed from the patient's body through a vein, and the white blood cells are separated from the rest of the blood components using a special machine. The stem cells are then frozen and stored until they are needed for reinfusion.

Following the collection of stem cells, the patient receives high-dose chemotherapy to kill the remaining leukemia cells. This chemotherapy is typically more intensive than the chemotherapy used for standard treatment. The goal of this approach is to completely eliminate the leukemia cells and reset the bone marrow so that it can produce healthy blood cells.

After the chemotherapy, the patient's frozen stem cells are thawed and reinfused back into the body. The stem cells then travel to the bone marrow, where they begin to produce new blood cells. It may take several weeks for the blood counts to return to normal levels.

Despite the advantages of autologous transplantation, it is not without risks. Patients undergoing autologous transplantation are at risk for infection and other complications related to the high-dose chemotherapy. Additionally, the success of the procedure depends on a variety of factors, including the patient's age, overall health, and the extent of the leukemia.

autologous stem cell transplantation is an important treatment option for patients with leukemia. The use of a patient's own stem cells allows for a reduced risk of rejection and other complications associated with transplantation. While the procedure is not without risks, it offers many benefits to patients who have undergone high-dose chemotherapy. As with any treatment for leukemia, patients should discuss the risks and benefits of autologous transplantation with their healthcare provider to determine if this approach is right for them.

Allogeneic Transplant

Allogeneic stem cell transplantation (allo-SCT) is a procedure in which stem cells are collected from a donor and transplanted into a patient with leukemia. This type of transplantation is different from autologous transplantation, in which the patient's own stem cells are collected and reinfused.

The goal of allo-SCT is to provide the patient with healthy stem cells that can produce normal blood cells and replace the abnormal ones that were causing the leukemia. The donor can be a family member or an unrelated individual who has a similar tissue type to the patient. The process of finding a suitable donor is called HLA typing.

1. There are two types of allo-SCT: myeloablative and non-myeloablative. Myeloablative transplantation involves the use of high-dose chemotherapy and/or radiation therapy to completely destroy the patient's bone marrow before the donor stem cells are infused. Non-myeloablative transplantation, also known as reduced-intensity conditioning, uses lower doses of chemotherapy and radiation to suppress the patient's immune system and make room for the donor cells.

One of the advantages of allo-SCT is the potential for graft-versus-leukemia (GVL) effect. This occurs when the donor's immune cells recognize and attack the patient's leukemia cells. This effect can be beneficial in eradicating the leukemia and preventing relapse.

However, allo-SCT also carries the risk of graft-versus-host disease (GVHD), a condition in which the donor immune cells attack the patient's normal tissues. GVHD can affect multiple organs and can be life-threatening. Therefore, patients receiving allo-SCT require close monitoring and treatment with immunosuppressive medications to prevent or manage GVHD.

The success of allo-SCT depends on several factors, including the patient's age and overall health, the stage and type of leukemia, the degree of HLA matching between the donor and recipient, and the type of conditioning regimen used. The overall survival rate for allo-SCT varies depending on these factors, but it is generally higher than that of chemotherapy alone.

allo-SCT is an important treatment option for patients with leukemia who are eligible for this procedure. It offers the potential for a cure through replacement of abnormal cells with healthy ones, as well as the benefit of GVL effect. However, it also carries the risk of GVHD and requires close monitoring and management. The success of allo-SCT depends on multiple factors and requires a multidisciplinary approach involving the patient, hematologist/oncologist, transplant team, and other healthcare professionals.

Preparative Regimens and Graft-Versus-Host Disease

Leukemia is a group of blood cancers that affect the production of blood cells in the bone marrow. It is a complex disease with many subtypes, each requiring a different approach to treatment. In cases where chemotherapy and radiation therapy are not effective, stem cell transplantation is often recommended. This procedure involves replacing the patient's diseased bone marrow with healthy cells from a donor. However, to prevent rejection of the new cells, the patient must undergo preparative regimens that can cause significant side effects, including graft-versus-host disease.

Preparative regimens are intensive treatments that are used to prepare a patient's body for a stem cell transplant. These regimens typically involve high doses of chemotherapy and/or radiation therapy, which are intended to destroy the patient's own bone marrow and immune system. The purpose of this is to make space in the patient's bone marrow for the new stem cells and to prevent the patient's immune system from rejecting them.

The specific preparative regimen used depends on several factors, including the type of leukemia, the patient's age and overall health, and the availability of a suitable donor. Generally, a more aggressive regimen is used for patients with high-risk leukemia or those who have had a relapse after previous treatments.

One of the main risks associated with preparative regimens is graft-versus-host disease (GVHD), which occurs when the transplanted cells recognize the patient's body as foreign and attack healthy tissues. GVHD can affect various organs and can range from mild to severe. The risk of developing GVHD is higher in allogeneic transplants, where the donor cells come from someone else, compared to autologous transplants, where the patient's own cells are used.

To reduce the risk of GVHD, patients may receive immunosuppressive drugs after the transplant. These drugs work by suppressing the activity of the immune system and reducing the likelihood of an attack on the patient's healthy tissues. However, this also makes the patient more susceptible to infections.

Other potential side effects of preparative regimens include nausea, vomiting, hair loss, and fatigue. Patients may also experience a decrease in their blood cell counts, which can lead to anemia, infections, and bleeding. These side effects are generally temporary and can be managed with medications and other supportive measures.

Despite the risks and potential side effects, stem cell transplantation can be a life-saving treatment for patients with leukemia who have exhausted other options. The success rate of the procedure depends on several factors, including the patient's age and overall health, the type of leukemia, and the compatibility of the donor cells.

preparative regimens are an essential part of the stem cell transplantation process for patients with leukemia. While they can cause significant side effects, they are necessary to prepare the patient's body for the transplant and reduce the risk of rejection. Patients undergoing a stem cell transplant should work closely with their healthcare team to manage the side effects and ensure the best possible outcome.

Immunotherapy

Immunotherapy is a promising treatment for leukemia that harnesses the power of the immune system to target and destroy cancer cells. Unlike chemotherapy and radiation, which target all rapidly dividing cells, including healthy ones, immunotherapy is more targeted and specifically focuses on cancer cells.

The immune system is the body's natural defense against infection and disease. It works by recognizing and attacking foreign substances, such as bacteria, viruses, and cancer cells. However, cancer cells are often able to evade the immune system's defenses and grow unchecked.

Immunotherapy aims to overcome this by boosting the immune system's ability to recognize and attack cancer cells. There are several types of immunotherapy currently being used to treat leukemia.

One type of immunotherapy is monoclonal antibodies. These are laboratory-made versions of natural immune system proteins that can be designed to specifically target cancer cells. When these antibodies bind to cancer cells, they can either signal the immune system to attack the cancer cells or deliver a toxic substance directly to the cancer cells.

Another type of immunotherapy is chimeric antigen receptor (CAR) T-cell therapy. This involves genetically modifying a patient's T-cells, a type of immune cell, to recognize and attack cancer cells. In CAR T-cell therapy, T-cells are extracted from a patient's blood and genetically engineered to produce a receptor that specifically targets a protein on the surface of leukemia cells. The modified T-cells are then infused back into the patient's body, where they can seek out and destroy cancer cells.

Another promising approach to immunotherapy is checkpoint inhibitors. Normally, checkpoint proteins help regulate the immune system by preventing it from attacking healthy cells. However, cancer cells can sometimes exploit these checkpoints to evade the immune system. Checkpoint inhibitors block these proteins, allowing the immune system to attack cancer cells more effectively.

One of the benefits of immunotherapy is that it can produce long-lasting remissions in some patients. However, it is not without risks. Like any treatment, immunotherapy can cause side effects, including fatigue, fever, and chills. More serious side effects can occur, including organ damage and autoimmune reactions.

It is important to note that immunotherapy is still a relatively new treatment for leukemia, and more research is needed to fully understand its potential benefits and risks. However, it has shown promise in clinical trials and is currently being used to treat certain types of leukemia.

immunotherapy is a promising treatment option for leukemia that aims to harness the power of the immune system to fight cancer. There are several types of immunotherapy currently being used, including monoclonal antibodies, CAR T-cell therapy, and checkpoint inhibitors. While immunotherapy has shown promise in clinical trials, more research is needed to fully understand its potential benefits and risks. Nonetheless, it represents an exciting area of research that has the potential to revolutionize the treatment of leukemia and other types of cancer.

Monoclonal Antibodies

Monoclonal antibodies (mAbs) are a type of immunotherapy that are used in the treatment of leukemia. mAbs are laboratory-made proteins that are designed to mimic the immune system's ability to fight off cancer cells. These antibodies can be engineered to target specific proteins on the surface of cancer cells, enabling them to bind to and destroy the cancer cells.

There are several types of monoclonal antibodies that have been approved for the treatment of leukemia, including rituximab, alemtuzumab, and blinatumomab. These antibodies have been shown to be effective in treating different types of leukemia and have revolutionized the treatment of this disease.

Rituximab is a monoclonal antibody that is used to treat B-cell non-Hodgkin's lymphoma and chronic lymphocytic leukemia. This antibody targets a protein called CD20, which is found on the surface of B-cells. When rituximab binds to CD20, it triggers an immune response that leads to the destruction of the cancer cells. Rituximab is typically used in combination with chemotherapy and has been shown to improve survival rates in patients with B-cell non-Hodgkin's lymphoma.

Alemtuzumab is a monoclonal antibody that is used to treat chronic lymphocytic leukemia. This antibody targets a protein called CD52, which is found on the surface of B-cells and T-cells. When alemtuzumab binds to CD52, it triggers an immune response that leads to the destruction of the cancer cells. Alemtuzumab is often used as a second-line treatment in patients who have not responded to other therapies.

Blinatumomab is a monoclonal antibody that is used to treat B-cell acute lymphoblastic leukemia. This antibody targets a protein called CD19, which is found on the surface of B-cells. When blinatumomab binds to CD19, it triggers an immune response that leads to the destruction of the cancer cells. Blinatumomab is used in patients who have relapsed or have not responded to other treatments.

Monoclonal antibodies have several advantages over traditional chemotherapy drugs. They are more specific in their targeting of cancer cells, which means they can destroy cancer cells while leaving healthy cells unharmed. They also have fewer side effects than chemotherapy drugs, which can cause nausea, hair loss, and other unpleasant symptoms.

However, monoclonal antibodies are not without their drawbacks. They can be expensive to produce and administer, and they may not work for all patients. Some patients may also develop resistance to monoclonal antibodies over time, which can limit their effectiveness.

In addition to their use in treating leukemia, monoclonal antibodies are also being studied as a potential treatment for other types of cancer. Researchers are exploring ways to use these antibodies to target specific proteins on the surface of cancer cells, which could lead to more effective and less toxic cancer treatments.

Overall, monoclonal antibodies have revolutionized the treatment of leukemia and have provided new hope for patients who were once considered incurable. As researchers continue to develop new and more effective therapies, it is likely that monoclonal antibodies will play an increasingly important role in the fight against cancer.

Adoptive Cell Therapy

Adoptive cell therapy (ACT) is an emerging form of immunotherapy that involves the transfer of autologous or allogeneic immune cells that have been specifically engineered to recognize and kill cancer cells. This promising approach has shown great potential for the treatment of various types of cancer, including leukemia.

Leukemia is a cancer of the blood and bone marrow that results in the abnormal production of white blood cells. There are several different subtypes of leukemia, including acute lymphoblastic leukemia (ALL), acute myeloid leukemia (AML), chronic lymphocytic leukemia (CLL), and chronic myeloid leukemia (CML). While the prognosis for leukemia has improved over the years, with the development of new treatments such as chemotherapy and stem cell transplantation, there is still a need for more effective and less toxic therapies.

ACT has the potential to provide a more targeted and less toxic approach to the treatment of leukemia. One approach to ACT involves the use of chimeric antigen receptor (CAR) T cells. CAR T cells are genetically engineered immune cells that are designed to target cancer cells. They are created by taking T cells, a type of immune cell that normally fights infection, from a patient's blood and modifying them to express a CAR on their surface.

The CAR is made up of an antibody-like structure that is designed to recognize a specific protein on the surface of cancer cells. When the CAR T cell encounters a cancer cell that expresses the targeted protein, it binds to the cancer cell and releases chemicals that trigger the destruction of the cancer cell.

CAR T cell therapy has shown promising results in the treatment of ALL and lymphoma, and has recently been approved for the treatment of certain types of leukemia. In clinical trials, CAR T cell therapy has been shown to induce complete remission in a significant percentage of patients with relapsed or refractory ALL.

Another approach to ACT involves the use of tumor-infiltrating lymphocytes (TILs). TILs are immune cells that have infiltrated a tumor and are capable of recognizing and attacking cancer cells. In TIL therapy, TILs are isolated from a patient's tumor, expanded in the laboratory, and then infused back into the patient.

While TIL therapy has shown promising results in the treatment of solid tumors, it has not yet been extensively studied in the treatment of leukemia. However, preclinical studies suggest that TIL therapy may be effective in the treatment of certain types of leukemia, particularly those that express specific proteins on their surface.

Another type of ACT that is being studied in the treatment of leukemia is natural killer (NK) cell therapy. NK cells are a type of immune cell that are capable of recognizing and killing cancer cells. In NK cell therapy, NK cells are isolated from a patient's blood or from a donor, and then infused back into the patient.

While NK cell therapy has shown promising results in preclinical studies, it has not yet been extensively studied in clinical trials for the treatment of leukemia. However, there is growing interest in the potential of NK cell therapy, particularly in combination with other therapies such as chemotherapy and CAR T cell therapy.

In addition to CAR T cell therapy, TIL therapy, and NK cell therapy, there are several other types of ACT that are being studied in the treatment of leukemia. These include T cell receptor (TCR) therapy, which involves the modification of T cells to recognize cancer-specific proteins, and dendritic cell therapy, which involves the stimulation of the patient's immune system to recognize and attack cancer cells.

Overall, ACT represents an exciting new approach to the treatment of leukemia. While much more research is needed to fully understand the potential of these therapies, early results suggest that they may provide a more targeted and less toxic approach to the treatment of this devastating disease.

Immune Checkpoint Inhibitors

Immune checkpoint inhibitors are a type of cancer treatment that is designed to help the immune system recognize and attack cancer cells. These inhibitors block certain molecules on cancer cells or immune cells, called checkpoints, that would normally keep the immune system from attacking cancer cells. By blocking these checkpoints, immune checkpoint inhibitors can help the immune system better recognize and attack cancer cells.

In the context of leukemia, immune checkpoint inhibitors have shown promising results in the treatment of certain types of leukemia. Leukemia is a type of cancer that affects the blood and bone marrow, and is characterized by the abnormal growth and proliferation of white blood cells. The immune system plays a crucial role in the development and progression of leukemia, and immune checkpoint inhibitors are a relatively new approach to leukemia treatment that target the immune system.

One of the most promising targets for immune checkpoint inhibitors in leukemia is the programmed death-ligand 1 (PD-L1) pathway. PD-L1 is a molecule that is expressed on the surface of many cancer cells, including leukemia cells, and interacts with another molecule on T cells called programmed cell death protein 1 (PD-1). This interaction inhibits the

T cells from attacking the cancer cells, allowing the cancer to grow and spread. Immune checkpoint inhibitors that block either PD-1 or PD-L1 can prevent this interaction, allowing the T cells to attack the cancer cells.

Several clinical trials have investigated the use of immune checkpoint inhibitors in the treatment of leukemia. For example, a phase I trial of the PD-1 inhibitor pembrolizumab in patients with relapsed or refractory acute myeloid leukemia (AML) showed promising results. In this trial, 36% of patients had a complete response or partial response to the treatment, and the response was durable in many of these patients. Another study investigated the use of the PD-L1 inhibitor atezolizumab in combination with chemotherapy in patients with AML. This study showed that the combination therapy was well-tolerated and had a high response rate.

In addition to PD-1 and PD-L1, other immune checkpoint molecules are also being investigated as targets for immune checkpoint inhibitors in leukemia. For example, the molecule CTLA-4 is another checkpoint molecule that inhibits T cell activity. A phase I trial of the CTLA-4 inhibitor ipilimumab in patients with relapsed or refractory AML showed that the treatment was safe and had some evidence of clinical activity.

While the use of immune checkpoint inhibitors in leukemia is still in the early stages of investigation, these therapies have shown promise in early clinical trials. However, there are also some challenges and limitations to the use of immune checkpoint inhibitors in leukemia. For example, not all patients with leukemia express high levels of PD-L1 or other checkpoint molecules, and the response rates to immune checkpoint inhibitors can be highly variable. Additionally, these therapies can cause immune-related adverse events, which can be serious or even life-threatening.

Overall, the development of immune checkpoint inhibitors as a treatment option for leukemia represents an exciting new approach to cancer therapy.

While there is still much to learn about the optimal use of these therapies in leukemia, early results are encouraging and suggest that immune checkpoint inhibitors may have an important role to play in the treatment of this disease.

Supportive Care

Leukemia, a cancer of the blood and bone marrow, can be a devastating disease that requires intensive treatment. In addition to aggressive therapies such as chemotherapy and stem cell transplantation, patients also require supportive care to manage symptoms and side effects of treatment. Supportive care is an important aspect of leukemia treatment and can improve patients' quality of life while undergoing therapy.

1. Supportive care can be divided into two main categories: symptom management and infection prevention. Symptoms of leukemia can vary depending on the type and stage of the disease but may include fatigue, fever, weight loss, anemia, and bleeding or bruising easily. These symptoms can be managed with medications such as pain relievers, anti-nausea drugs, and blood transfusions.

Fatigue is a common symptom of leukemia and can be managed through lifestyle changes such as increasing physical activity, eating a balanced diet, and getting adequate rest. Exercise has been shown to reduce fatigue in cancer patients and can also improve overall physical function and quality of life.

In addition to managing symptoms, preventing infections is critical for patients with leukemia. Chemotherapy and other treatments can weaken the immune system, making patients more vulnerable to infections. Infections can be serious and even life-threatening for patients with leukemia, so prevention measures are critical.

Patients with leukemia may receive prophylactic antibiotics to prevent infections or may be instructed to avoid contact with individuals who have recently been ill or who have known infections. Patients may also receive vaccinations to prevent certain infections, such as pneumonia or the flu. Hand hygiene and other infection control practices are also important for preventing the spread of infection.

Nutrition is another important aspect of supportive care for patients with leukemia. Chemotherapy and radiation therapy can cause side effects such as nausea, vomiting, and loss of appetite, which can make it difficult to consume enough nutrients. Proper nutrition is important for maintaining strength and energy levels, as well as for supporting the immune system.

Registered dietitians can work with patients to develop a balanced diet that meets their individual needs and preferences. In some cases, patients may require enteral or parenteral nutrition, which involves providing nutrients directly into the bloodstream or gastrointestinal tract.

Psychological support is also an important component of supportive care for patients with leukemia. A cancer diagnosis can be overwhelming and emotional, and patients may experience anxiety, depression, or other psychological symptoms. Support from family, friends, and healthcare professionals can help patients cope with the emotional impact of leukemia and its treatment.

Psychological interventions such as cognitive-behavioral therapy, mindfulness-based stress reduction, and support groups have been shown to improve quality of life and reduce psychological distress in cancer patients.

supportive care is an essential part of leukemia treatment. Symptom management, infection prevention, nutrition, and psychological support are all important components of supportive care for patients with leukemia. A multidisciplinary approach that includes healthcare professionals from various disciplines can provide the most comprehensive and effective supportive care for patients with leukemia.

Blood Transfusions

Blood transfusions are a vital part of supportive care for patients with leukemia, a type of cancer that affects the blood and bone marrow. Leukemia can cause low blood counts, leading to anemia, infections, and bleeding problems. Transfusions of blood and blood products can help address these issues and improve the quality of life for leukemia patients.

Blood transfusions involve transferring blood or blood products from a donor to a recipient. The most common type of transfusion is a red blood cell transfusion, which provides oxygen-carrying red blood cells to replace those that have been lost due to bleeding or destruction by chemotherapy. Platelet transfusions, which provide blood-clotting cells, are also frequently used in leukemia patients who are at risk of bleeding due to low platelet counts. Additionally, some patients may require transfusions of plasma, which contains clotting factors, or other blood products such as albumin or immunoglobulins.

1. Before a transfusion, a patient's blood type and the compatibility of the donor's blood must be determined to avoid complications such as hemolysis, a potentially life-threatening reaction in which the recipient's immune system attacks and destroys the transfused red blood cells. Blood typing is typically done using the ABO system, which classifies blood into four types: A, B, AB, and O. Each type is further characterized by the presence or absence of the Rh factor, resulting in eight possible blood types.

Blood transfusions carry some risks, such as transfusion reactions, infections, and transfusion-related lung injury, but these risks are generally low with modern blood banking practices. Patients receiving transfusions are monitored closely for any signs of adverse reactions, such as fever, chills, itching, or breathing difficulties.

In addition to blood transfusions, supportive care for leukemia patients may include medications to stimulate the production of blood cells, antibiotics to prevent or treat infections, and growth factors to boost the immune system. Pain management and emotional support are also important aspects of supportive care for patients with leukemia.

Patients with leukemia may require multiple blood transfusions throughout their treatment course. The frequency and duration of transfusions depend on the patient's disease stage, treatment regimen, and individual response. Transfusions may be given on an as-needed basis to address specific symptoms or on a regular schedule to maintain adequate blood counts.

One potential complication of frequent blood transfusions is iron overload, which can occur when the body accumulates excess iron from transfused red blood cells. Iron overload can damage organs such as the liver, heart, and pancreas and can lead to conditions such as diabetes, heart failure, and liver disease. To prevent or treat iron overload, patients may receive chelation therapy, which involves using medications to remove excess iron from the body.

blood transfusions are an important part of supportive care for leukemia patients. They provide a means of addressing low blood counts and associated symptoms, such as anemia and bleeding problems. Although there are risks associated with transfusions, these risks are generally low with modern blood banking practices. Patients with leukemia may require multiple transfusions throughout their treatment course, and monitoring for potential complications such as iron overload is an important aspect of supportive care. Ultimately, the goal of supportive care is to improve the quality of life for leukemia patients and optimize their response to treatment.

Infection Prevention and Management

Leukemia is a type of cancer that affects the blood and bone marrow, leading to the production of abnormal white blood cells. The condition weakens the immune system and increases the risk of infections. Hence, infection prevention and management are essential for patients with leukemia.

Infection Prevention:

Infection prevention measures aim to reduce the risk of infection in leukemia patients. This includes taking precautions to prevent exposure to infectious agents, such as bacteria, viruses, and fungi. Patients with leukemia have a compromised immune system, making them more susceptible to infections. Hence, it is vital to follow strict hygiene measures, such as washing hands frequently, avoiding contact with sick people, and maintaining a clean environment.

Immunization is another important infection prevention measure. Patients with leukemia are at increased risk of infections, and vaccination can help prevent infections such as influenza, pneumonia, and hepatitis. However, leukemia patients may not respond well to vaccines due to their compromised immune system. Hence, vaccination should be done before the diagnosis of leukemia, if possible.

Infection Management:

Despite taking preventive measures, patients with leukemia may still develop infections. The management of infections in leukemia patients is crucial, as untreated infections can lead to severe complications and even death.

Prompt recognition and diagnosis of infection are crucial for effective management. Common signs of infection include fever, chills, fatigue, and coughing. If an infection is suspected, the patient should undergo diagnostic tests, such as blood cultures, urine cultures, and imaging studies.

Antibiotic therapy is the mainstay of infection management in leukemia patients. The choice of antibiotics depends on the type of infection and the patient's clinical condition. Antibiotics should be started promptly and administered for the recommended duration to avoid the development of antibiotic resistance.

In some cases, antifungal and antiviral therapies may be required, especially in patients with prolonged neutropenia. Neutropenia is a condition where the number of white blood cells is abnormally low, leaving the body vulnerable to infections.

In addition to pharmacological therapy, supportive care measures are also crucial in managing infections in leukemia patients. This includes measures such as maintaining adequate hydration, pain management, and nutritional support. In severe cases, hospitalization may be required for intravenous antibiotics, fluid and electrolyte management, and close monitoring.

Infection prevention and management are essential in the care of leukemia patients. Preventive measures, such as strict hygiene and immunization, aim to reduce the risk of infections, while prompt recognition and diagnosis of infections are crucial for effective management. Antibiotic therapy, along with supportive care measures, is the mainstay of infection management in leukemia patients. By taking these measures, the risk of infections can be minimized, and the outcome of leukemia treatment can be improved.

Clinical trials for Leukemia patients

Clinical trials are research studies designed to find new and innovative ways to diagnose, prevent, or treat a disease such as Leukemia. These studies may involve testing new drugs, procedures, or medical devices. Clinical trials are an essential part of the medical research process and can help improve patient outcomes and quality of life.

Leukemia patients may be eligible to participate in clinical trials if they meet certain criteria. Patients may consider participating in clinical trials if they have not responded to standard treatments or if they are seeking new treatment options. Patients can talk to their healthcare providers to see if they are eligible for any ongoing clinical trials.

Clinical trials can be divided into four phases:

Phase I trials are the first step in testing a new treatment in humans. They are designed to evaluate the safety of the treatment and determine the appropriate dosage.

Phase II trials involve a larger group of patients and are designed to evaluate the effectiveness of the treatment and further assess its safety.

Phase III trials are larger studies that compare the new treatment with the standard treatment to determine which is more effective.

Phase IV trials are conducted after a treatment has been approved and are designed to monitor its long-term safety and effectiveness.

Participating in a clinical trial can have its risks and benefits. Patients should talk to their healthcare providers and do their own research to weigh the risks and benefits of participating in a clinical trial.

In conclusion, clinical trials are a valuable part of the research process and can offer new treatment options for Leukemia patients. Patients should talk to their healthcare providers to see if they are eligible for any ongoing clinical trials.

Types of Clinical Trials

Clinical trials are scientific studies conducted to evaluate the safety and effectiveness of new medical treatments, procedures, and interventions. They are essential for discovering new therapies that can potentially benefit patients with various diseases, including leukemia. Clinical trials come in different types, each with its own specific objective and design. In this essay, we will explore the different types of clinical trials and their relevance to leukemia treatment.

1. Phase 0 Trials: Phase 0 trials are also known as exploratory trials or micro-dose trials. They are the first step in the clinical trial process and involve testing very low doses of an experimental drug or treatment on a small number of participants. These trials are used to determine if the drug behaves in the way it was designed to and if it has any potential therapeutic benefits. Phase 0 trials are not typically used for leukemia treatment.

2. Phase I Trials: Phase I trials are the next step in the clinical trial process and involve testing the safety and tolerability of an experimental drug or treatment. These trials are conducted on a small number of patients who

have advanced leukemia and have exhausted all other treatment options. The primary objective of a Phase I trial is to determine the maximum tolerated dose of the drug and to evaluate any adverse effects. Phase I trials are essential for establishing the safety profile of a drug or treatment before moving to larger trials.

3. Phase II Trials: Phase II trials are conducted on a larger group of patients than Phase I trials, typically between 20-100 participants. These trials are designed to evaluate the effectiveness of the drug or treatment in treating the disease. In leukemia, Phase II trials may involve comparing a new drug or combination of drugs to an existing standard of care. The primary objective of a Phase II trial is to determine if the treatment is effective in slowing or stopping the progression of leukemia.

4. Phase III Trials: Phase III trials are the final step in the clinical trial process and involve testing the effectiveness and safety of a new treatment in comparison to the standard of care. These trials involve large numbers of patients, often in the thousands, and can take several years to complete. In leukemia, Phase III trials may involve comparing a new drug or treatment to the current standard of care, such as chemotherapy or stem cell transplantation. The primary objective of a Phase III trial is to determine if the new treatment is more effective and safer than the standard of care.

5. Phase IV Trials: Phase IV trials are conducted after a drug or treatment has been approved by regulatory agencies and is available to the public. These trials are designed to monitor the long-term safety and effectiveness of the drug or treatment in a larger population. In leukemia, Phase IV trials may involve monitoring the effectiveness of a new drug or treatment in real-world settings, outside of a controlled clinical trial.

6. Randomized Controlled Trials: Randomized controlled trials are the gold standard for clinical trials and involve randomly assigning patients to

either the experimental group or the control group. In leukemia, randomized controlled trials may involve comparing a new drug or treatment to a placebo or an existing standard of care. Randomized controlled trials are essential for ensuring that the results of a clinical trial are not influenced by bias.

7. Non-Randomized Trials: Non-randomized trials do not involve randomly assigning patients to a treatment group. Instead, patients may self-select or be assigned to a group based on their disease characteristics or other factors. Non-randomized trials are generally less reliable than randomized controlled trials, but they can still provide valuable information about the safety and effectiveness of a treatment.

clinical trials are an essential component of leukemia treatment and research. Each type of clinical trial has a specific objective and design, and they are all important for discovering new therapies and improving the outcomes of leukemia patients. As the field of leukemia research continues to evolve, clinical trials will continue to play a critical role in developing new treatments and improving the standard of care.

Benefits and Risks

Clinical trials are an essential part of the research and development process for new medical treatments, and they play a critical role in the fight against leukemia. The benefits and risks of participating in clinical trials are important considerations for patients and their healthcare providers.

Clinical trials offer numerous potential benefits for leukemia patients. First and foremost, clinical trials provide access to new and innovative treatments that may not be available through standard care. These treatments may be more effective, less toxic, or have fewer side effects than existing therapies. In some cases, clinical trials may also offer the opportunity for patients to receive treatment that is personalized to their specific disease or genetic profile.

Another potential benefit of participating in clinical trials is the opportunity to receive more frequent and intensive medical monitoring. Patients in clinical trials typically receive close attention from their healthcare team, with more frequent check-ups, lab tests, and imaging scans. This can be especially important for leukemia patients who may need regular monitoring to ensure their disease is responding to treatment or to detect any potential complications.

In addition to the potential benefits, there are also risks associated with participating in clinical trials. One of the primary risks is the possibility of experiencing side effects or complications from the experimental treatment. Because these treatments are often new and untested, their safety profile may not be fully understood. This means that patients may be at risk for side effects that are not yet known or may be more severe than expected.

Another potential risk of clinical trials is the possibility of receiving a placebo or ineffective treatment. In some cases, clinical trials may use a control group that receives a placebo or standard treatment instead of the experimental therapy. This is done to compare the effectiveness of the new treatment to the standard of care. However, it means that patients in the control group may not receive the potentially life-saving benefits of the new treatment.

Finally, participating in clinical trials may require a significant time commitment and may involve travel or other logistical challenges. This can be especially difficult for leukemia patients who may already be dealing with the physical and emotional toll of their disease and treatment.

Despite the risks, many leukemia patients and their healthcare providers believe that the potential benefits of clinical trials outweigh the potential risks. It is important for patients to carefully consider their options and discuss the potential risks and benefits with their healthcare team before making a decision about whether to participate in a clinical trial.

clinical trials are a vital part of the fight against leukemia, offering new and innovative treatments that may improve patient outcomes. However, they also carry potential risks and require careful consideration before making a decision to participate. Patients and their healthcare providers must weigh the potential benefits against the risks and make an informed decision based on the individual patient's needs and circumstances.

Participating in Clinical Trials

Clinical trials are an essential aspect of medical research and play a crucial role in advancing our understanding and treatment of various diseases, including leukemia. Leukemia is a type of cancer that affects the blood and bone marrow, and it requires careful treatment planning and management to achieve the best possible outcomes. Participating in clinical trials can provide several benefits for leukemia patients, but it is important to understand the risks and make an informed decision about whether to participate.

One of the primary benefits of participating in a clinical trial is the access to new and innovative treatments that may not be available through standard treatment options. Clinical trials are designed to test new drugs, therapies, and procedures that may offer improved outcomes for leukemia patients. These treatments are typically not yet approved by regulatory agencies like the FDA, but they have shown promising results in earlier stages of research.

In addition to access to new treatments, participating in clinical trials also provides an opportunity to receive a higher level of care and monitoring. Patients who participate in clinical trials are closely monitored by a team of medical professionals who specialize in their condition. This level of care can help detect any side effects or complications early on and provide prompt intervention to manage them effectively.

Clinical trials can also be a source of hope for leukemia patients and their families. Many clinical trials are designed to test treatments that have the potential to be more effective than standard treatments, or to provide new options for patients who have not responded to other treatments. Participating in a clinical trial can give patients a sense of empowerment and control over their disease, as well as a sense of contributing to the advancement of medical research.

Despite the potential benefits of clinical trials, there are also risks associated with participating. These risks can include side effects or complications from the treatment, as well as the possibility that the treatment may not be effective. Patients who participate in clinical trials must also undergo additional testing and monitoring, which can be time-consuming and may require additional travel to medical facilities.

It is important for patients to carefully consider the potential risks and benefits of participating in a clinical trial before making a decision. Patients should discuss their options with their healthcare provider and carefully review the informed consent documents provided by the clinical trial sponsor. Informed consent documents should provide detailed information about the study's purpose, design, treatment options, and potential risks and benefits.

Patients who decide to participate in a clinical trial must also be committed to following the study's protocol and attending all required appointments and follow-up visits. Patients who do not adhere to the study protocol may be asked to withdraw from the trial, which can impact their treatment options.

To participate in a clinical trial, patients must meet certain eligibility criteria. These criteria may include factors such as age, overall health, and specific disease characteristics. Patients who are interested in participating in a clinical trial should talk to their healthcare provider about their eligibility and any potential barriers to participation.

clinical trials play a critical role in advancing our understanding and treatment of leukemia. Participating in a clinical trial can provide access to new treatments, a higher level of care and monitoring, and a sense of hope for patients and their families. However, it is important to carefully consider the potential risks and benefits of participating before making a decision. Patients who are interested in participating in a clinical trial should talk to their healthcare provider and review the informed consent documents provided by the clinical trial sponsor to make an informed decision about whether to participate.

Pediatric Leukemia

Leukemia is a type of cancer that affects the blood and bone marrow, and it is the most common cancer in children. In pediatric leukemia, the cancerous cells are produced in the bone marrow and spread into the blood, affecting the white blood cells, which are responsible for fighting infections. Childhood leukemia can be classified into two main types: acute lymphoblastic leukemia (ALL) and acute myeloid leukemia (AML).

Acute lymphoblastic leukemia (ALL) is the most common type of pediatric leukemia, accounting for about 80% of cases. It occurs when the bone marrow produces too many immature white blood cells, which are called lymphoblasts. These immature cells can't function properly and crowd out the normal, healthy blood cells. ALL can develop quickly and can be life-threatening if not treated promptly.

Acute myeloid leukemia (AML) is less common than ALL, but it is still a significant health concern. AML occurs when the bone marrow produces too many immature myeloid cells, which are another type of white blood cell. These cells can also interfere with the production of healthy blood cells, leading to anemia, infection, and bleeding.

The exact cause of pediatric leukemia is unknown, but several factors have been identified as potential risk factors. These include exposure to radiation, certain chemicals, and genetic factors. Children with certain genetic disorders, such as Down syndrome, have an increased risk of developing leukemia.

The symptoms of pediatric leukemia can vary depending on the type of leukemia and the stage of the disease. Common symptoms include:

- Fatigue
- Weakness
- Pale skin
- Shortness of breath
- Easy bruising or bleeding
- Fever
- Infections that don't go away or keep coming back
- Pain in the bones or joints

- Swollen lymph nodes

Diagnosis of pediatric leukemia usually begins with a physical exam and a review of the child's medical history. The doctor will then order a series of tests to confirm the diagnosis, including blood tests, bone marrow aspiration and biopsy, and imaging tests such as x-rays, CT scans, and MRI.

Once a diagnosis of leukemia is confirmed, the child will undergo further tests to determine the subtype and the stage of the disease. This information is crucial in determining the appropriate treatment options.

Treatment for pediatric leukemia usually involves a combination of chemotherapy, radiation therapy, and sometimes a stem cell transplant. Chemotherapy involves the use of drugs to kill cancer cells, while radiation therapy uses high-energy radiation to kill cancer cells. A stem cell transplant involves replacing the child's bone marrow with healthy stem cells to restore the body's ability to produce healthy blood cells.

The specific treatment plan will depend on several factors, including the type and stage of leukemia, the child's age and overall health, and the family's preferences. It is essential to discuss all treatment options with the child's medical team and to carefully consider the potential benefits and risks of each option.

In addition to medical treatment, supportive care is crucial in managing the side effects of treatment and improving the child's quality of life. Supportive care may include pain management, infection prevention and management, blood transfusions, and nutritional support.

Participating in clinical trials is another important option for children with leukemia. Clinical trials involve testing new treatments or procedures to determine their safety and effectiveness. Participating in a clinical trial can provide access to new and potentially more effective treatments, but it is important to carefully consider the potential benefits and risks before enrolling in a trial.

pediatric leukemia is a serious and potentially life-threatening disease, but advances in medical treatment have greatly improved the outlook for children with this condition.

Unique Characteristics

Leukemia is a type of cancer that affects the blood and bone marrow, and it can develop in anyone regardless of age, gender, or ethnicity. However, there are some unique characteristics of leukemia that make it different from other types of cancer. In this essay, we will explore these characteristics and what makes leukemia so unique.

1. One of the unique characteristics of leukemia is its classification system. Leukemia is classified based on the type of blood cells affected and the rate of cell growth. There are four main types of leukemia: acute lymphoblastic leukemia (ALL), acute myeloid leukemia (AML), chronic lymphocytic leukemia (CLL), and chronic myeloid leukemia (CML). These types are further classified based on the cell characteristics and other factors. The World Health Organization (WHO) classification system is widely used to categorize leukemia, and it takes into account genetic and molecular factors that affect the disease's behavior and treatment options.

Another unique characteristic of leukemia is that it can have a rapid onset and progression. Acute leukemias such as ALL and AML can develop rapidly and require immediate treatment, while chronic leukemias such as CLL and CML can develop slowly and may not require immediate intervention. The rapid onset of acute leukemia can make it challenging to diagnose, and immediate treatment is often necessary to prevent the disease from spreading.

Leukemia is also unique because it affects the blood and bone marrow, which are essential components of the body's immune system. Leukemia cells can interfere with the production of healthy blood cells, causing anemia, infection, and bleeding. This can weaken the immune system and increase the risk of infection and other complications. Additionally, leukemia can cause abnormal immune system activity, resulting in autoimmune disorders, where the body's immune system attacks its tissues and organs.

The treatment of leukemia is also unique, and it often involves a combination of different therapies, including chemotherapy, radiation therapy, stem cell transplantation, and immunotherapy. The treatment options depend on the type and stage of leukemia and the patient's overall health. Leukemia treatments can also have side effects such as nausea, hair loss, and fatigue, which can affect a patient's quality of life.

Another unique characteristic of leukemia is its impact on pediatric patients. Childhood leukemia is the most common cancer in children and accounts for approximately 30% of all childhood cancer cases. The symptoms and treatment of leukemia in children can be different from adults, and pediatric patients require specialized care and attention. Treatment options for pediatric leukemia may include chemotherapy, radiation therapy, and stem cell transplantation.

Leukemia also has a unique impact on the emotional and psychological well-being of patients and their families. A leukemia diagnosis can be overwhelming and stressful, and it can affect a patient's mental health and quality of life. Patients and their families may experience anxiety, depression, and social isolation, which can affect their ability to cope with the disease and the treatment.

leukemia is a unique type of cancer that affects the blood and bone marrow and can have a rapid onset and progression. The classification system, impact on the immune system, and treatment options for leukemia are also unique. Pediatric leukemia and the emotional and psychological impact of leukemia on patients and their families are additional unique characteristics of this disease. Despite the challenges, advances in leukemia research and treatment have improved patient outcomes and quality of life. It is essential to continue to support leukemia research and develop new therapies to improve treatment options for patients.

Treatment Approaches

Leukemia is a type of cancer that affects the blood and bone marrow, and it is characterized by the abnormal production of white blood cells. It is a complex disease, and its treatment often involves a combination of approaches. There are different treatment approaches that can be used to manage leukemia, and these approaches can be broadly classified into three categories: chemotherapy, radiation therapy, and immunotherapy. The choice of treatment approach will depend on various factors, including the type and stage of leukemia, the patient's age and overall health, and the patient's preferences.

Chemotherapy is a common treatment approach for leukemia, and it involves the use of drugs to kill cancer cells. Chemotherapy drugs can be administered orally or intravenously, and they work by disrupting the growth and division of cancer cells. The drugs used in chemotherapy are usually given in cycles, with rest periods in between to allow the body to recover from the effects of the drugs. Chemotherapy can cause side effects, such as hair loss, nausea, and fatigue, but these can be managed with medication and other supportive care measures.

Radiation therapy is another treatment approach for leukemia, and it involves the use of high-energy radiation to kill cancer cells. Radiation therapy can be administered externally or internally, and it is often used in combination with chemotherapy. External beam radiation therapy involves directing radiation from outside the body towards the cancerous cells, while internal radiation therapy involves inserting a radioactive source into the body near the cancerous cells. Like chemotherapy, radiation therapy can cause side effects, such as skin irritation and fatigue.

Immunotherapy is a newer treatment approach that has shown promise in treating leukemia. Immunotherapy works by harnessing the body's own immune system to fight cancer. There are different types of immunotherapy, including monoclonal antibodies, CAR-T cell therapy, and checkpoint inhibitors. Monoclonal antibodies are laboratory-made molecules that can recognize and bind to specific cancer cells, while CAR-T cell therapy involves removing immune cells from the patient's body, modifying them in a laboratory to recognize and attack cancer cells, and then infusing them back into the patient's body. Checkpoint inhibitors, on the other hand, work by blocking certain proteins on cancer cells that prevent the immune system from recognizing and attacking them.

In addition to these treatment approaches, there are also supportive care measures that can be used to manage the symptoms of leukemia and improve the patient's quality of life. Supportive care measures may include blood transfusions to replace red blood cells and platelets, antibiotics to treat infections, and pain management medications. These measures can help manage the side effects of treatment and improve the patient's overall well-being.

The choice of treatment approach for leukemia will depend on various factors, including the type and stage of the disease, the patient's age and overall health, and the patient's preferences. For example, older patients may not be able to tolerate the side effects of chemotherapy or radiation therapy, and may prefer a less invasive approach such as immunotherapy. Similarly, patients with certain types of leukemia may be better candidates for specific treatment approaches. For instance, patients with acute lymphoblastic leukemia (ALL) may benefit from CAR-T cell therapy, while those with chronic lymphocytic leukemia (CLL) may benefit from monoclonal antibodies.

leukemia is a complex disease that requires a multifaceted approach to treatment. Chemotherapy, radiation therapy, and immunotherapy are the main treatment approaches used to manage leukemia, and the choice of approach will depend on various factors, including the type and stage of the disease, the patient's age and overall health, and the patient's preferences. Supportive care measures can also be used to manage the symptoms of leukemia and improve the patient's quality of life. The development of new treatment approaches, such as immunotherapy, has brought hope.

Alternative treatments for

Leukemia

It is important to note that there is no scientific evidence to support the effectiveness of alternative treatments for Leukemia. While some patients may choose to use complementary and alternative therapies in conjunction with conventional medical treatments, it is important to discuss these options with a healthcare provider before beginning any treatment plan.

Some alternative treatments that have been used for Leukemia include:

Acupuncture: a traditional Chinese medicine practice that involves the insertion of thin needles into the skin at specific points to promote healing.

Herbal supplements: some herbs, such as echinacea and ginseng, have been used to boost the immune system and promote healing. However, it is important to note that herbs can have negative interactions with chemotherapy and other medications.

Massage therapy: a form of bodywork that involves the manipulation of muscles and soft tissues to promote relaxation and pain relief.

Yoga: a practice that combines physical postures, breathing exercises, and meditation to promote relaxation and reduce stress.

Meditation: a practice that involves focusing the mind on a specific object, thought, or activity to promote relaxation and reduce stress.

While these alternative treatments may provide some relief for patients, they are not a substitute for conventional medical treatments for Leukemia. It is important for patients to work with a healthcare provider to develop a comprehensive treatment plan that meets their individual needs and preferences.

What is the prognosis for

Leukemia

The prognosis for Leukemia depends on several factors, such as the type of Leukemia, age, overall health, and response to treatment. Some types of Leukemia, such as chronic lymphocytic Leukemia (CLL), progress slowly and may not require immediate treatment, while others, such as acute myelogenous Leukemia (AML), progress quickly and require more aggressive treatment.

With advances in treatment options, the prognosis for Leukemia has improved over the years. The five-year survival rate for all types of Leukemia is around 65%, but this varies widely depending on the type of Leukemia and other individual factors.

For acute Leukemia, the prognosis is generally poorer, with a five-year survival rate of around 25-40%. However, many patients can achieve remission with treatment and may live for several years or more.

For chronic Leukemia, the prognosis is generally better, with a five-year survival rate of around 80-90%. Some patients with chronic Leukemia can live for many years without requiring treatment.

It's important to note that each person's case is unique, and individual factors can greatly influence the prognosis. Close monitoring and ongoing treatment may be necessary to manage the disease and maintain the best possible quality of life.

Long-Term Effects and Follow-Up Care

Leukemia is a type of cancer that affects the blood and bone marrow, leading to the production of abnormal white blood cells. While treatment for leukemia is aimed at eradicating the cancer cells, it is important to consider the long-term effects of treatment and the need for follow-up care to ensure that the patient remains healthy and cancer-free. This essay will explore the long-term effects of leukemia treatment and the importance of follow-up care.

One of the most common long-term effects of leukemia treatment is the increased risk of infections. Chemotherapy and radiation therapy can weaken the immune system, making it more susceptible to infections. Patients may also be more prone to developing other types of cancers, such as lymphoma or solid tumors, due to the damage caused to healthy cells during treatment.

Another potential long-term effect of leukemia treatment is damage to organs such as the heart, lungs, liver, and kidneys. This can be caused by chemotherapy drugs or radiation therapy. The severity of organ damage can vary depending on the type and length of treatment, as well as the patient's overall health.

Patients who undergo stem cell transplantation may also experience graft-versus-host disease (GVHD), where the transplanted cells attack the patient's healthy cells. This can lead to a variety of symptoms, such as skin rashes, gastrointestinal issues, and liver problems. GVHD can occur immediately after transplantation or several months later, and may require ongoing treatment.

In addition to the physical effects of treatment, leukemia survivors may also experience emotional and psychological effects. Many patients may feel anxious, depressed, or experience post-traumatic stress disorder (PTSD) due to their cancer diagnosis and treatment. This can impact their quality of life and may require counseling or other forms of support.

Follow-up care is essential for monitoring the long-term effects of leukemia treatment and ensuring that any issues are identified and addressed promptly. Patients should undergo regular blood tests to monitor their blood counts and check for any signs of relapse. Imaging tests may also be performed to monitor organ function and check for any new tumors.

It is important for patients to maintain a healthy lifestyle after treatment, including a balanced diet and regular exercise. Patients should also avoid smoking and excessive alcohol consumption, which can increase the risk of developing other health issues.

Follow-up care may also involve regular check-ins with a medical team, including an oncologist, hematologist, or other specialists. These professionals can monitor the patient's progress and address any concerns or issues that arise. Patients may also be referred to a survivorship program, which can provide additional support and resources for managing the long-term effects of treatment.

while leukemia treatment is aimed at eradicating cancer cells, it is important to consider the potential long-term effects of treatment and the need for follow-up care. Patients may experience physical, emotional, and psychological effects of treatment, including infections, organ damage, and PTSD. Follow-up care is essential for monitoring these effects and ensuring that any issues are addressed promptly. Patients should maintain a healthy lifestyle and work closely with their medical team to manage the long-term effects of treatment and promote their overall health and well-being.

Research and Future Directions

Leukemia is a type of cancer that affects the blood and bone marrow, and can be a life-threatening disease if not treated promptly and appropriately. The current treatment options for leukemia include chemotherapy, radiation therapy, stem cell transplantation, immunotherapy, and targeted therapy. Despite the advances made in leukemia treatment, the disease still poses a significant challenge, especially in terms of treatment resistance, relapse, and long-term side effects. Therefore, there is a need for continuous research and development of new and improved therapies to combat this disease.

Research on leukemia has come a long way, and there are promising new therapies and approaches being developed. One area of research that has shown great potential is the use of targeted therapies. These therapies work by specifically targeting the cancer cells while sparing the healthy cells, reducing the toxicity and side effects associated with traditional chemotherapy.

One such targeted therapy is venetoclax, which is approved for use in patients with chronic lymphocytic leukemia (CLL). Venetoclax works by blocking a protein called B-cell lymphoma-2 (BCL-2), which is essential for the survival of cancer cells. By inhibiting BCL-2, venetoclax can induce apoptosis (programmed cell death) in cancer cells, leading to their destruction.

Another promising approach is the use of chimeric antigen receptor (CAR) T-cell therapy. This therapy involves genetically engineering the patient's T-cells to recognize and destroy cancer cells. The T-cells are modified to express a chimeric antigen receptor, which is designed to target a specific protein on the surface of cancer cells. Once the T-cells are re-infused into the patient's body, they can selectively target and destroy the cancer cells.

In addition to these targeted therapies, researchers are also exploring new immunotherapies for leukemia treatment. One such therapy is the use of checkpoint inhibitors. Checkpoint inhibitors work by blocking proteins that prevent the immune system from attacking cancer cells. By blocking these proteins, checkpoint inhibitors can unleash the immune system to attack and destroy cancer cells.

Aside from the development of new therapies, there is also research being done to improve the accuracy and precision of current treatments. For example, researchers are exploring the use of liquid biopsies to monitor treatment response and detect disease recurrence. Liquid biopsies involve analyzing the DNA, RNA, and proteins in a patient's blood to detect cancer cells or fragments of cancer cells. This approach can help detect relapse earlier than traditional imaging methods, allowing for earlier intervention and potentially improving outcomes.

Another area of research is focused on understanding the genetic and molecular mechanisms that drive leukemia development and progression. By understanding these mechanisms, researchers hope to identify new therapeutic targets and develop more effective treatments.

In addition to these approaches, there is also ongoing research into improving the supportive care and quality of life for leukemia patients. For example, researchers are exploring the use of mindfulness-based interventions, such as meditation and yoga, to help reduce stress, anxiety, and depression in leukemia patients.

Overall, research in leukemia is a constantly evolving field, with new discoveries and breakthroughs being made all the time. As researchers continue to work towards a cure for leukemia, the ultimate goal is to develop more effective, less toxic, and better-tolerated therapies that can improve the outcomes and quality of life for leukemia patients.

Advances in Leukemia Research

Leukemia is a type of cancer that affects the blood and bone marrow, and it is characterized by the uncontrolled growth of abnormal white blood cells. It is the most common type of cancer in children and the most diagnosed leukemia in adults is acute myeloid leukemia (AML). While leukemia can be treated through chemotherapy, radiation therapy, and stem cell transplants, there is still much research being done to advance treatment options and ultimately find a cure.

One of the major recent advances in leukemia research has been the development of targeted therapies. Traditional chemotherapy works by killing rapidly dividing cells, but it also affects healthy cells in the body. Targeted therapies, on the other hand, aim to specifically target cancer cells, minimizing harm to healthy cells. For example, tyrosine kinase inhibitors

(TKIs) have been developed to target specific genetic mutations found in some leukemias, such as chronic myeloid leukemia (CML). These drugs have been shown to be highly effective in treating CML and have led to improved survival rates.

Another area of research in leukemia is immunotherapy, which uses the body's own immune system to fight cancer. One type of immunotherapy that has shown promise in treating leukemia is CAR T-cell therapy. In this treatment, T-cells (a type of immune cell) are extracted from a patient's blood, modified to target cancer cells, and then reinfused into the patient. CAR T-cell therapy has been shown to be highly effective in treating certain types of leukemia, including acute lymphoblastic leukemia (ALL) and diffuse large B-cell lymphoma.

Advancements in genetic sequencing technology have also led to a greater understanding of the genetic mutations that cause leukemia. This knowledge has allowed researchers to develop more personalized treatment options for patients based on their specific genetic profile. For example, a study published in the New England Journal of Medicine found that patients with AML who received targeted therapy based on their genetic profile had a higher rate of complete remission and longer overall survival than those who received standard chemotherapy.

Research into leukemia also includes studies on the long-term effects of treatment. While treatments such as chemotherapy and radiation therapy can be effective in treating leukemia, they can also cause long-term side effects such as secondary cancers, heart disease, and infertility. Research is being done to develop treatments that minimize these side effects and improve the quality of life for leukemia survivors.

In addition to medical research, there is also a focus on improving supportive care for leukemia patients. This includes developing interventions to manage symptoms such as pain, fatigue, and depression, as well as providing emotional and psychological support to patients and their families.

The field of leukemia research is constantly evolving, with new treatments and discoveries being made every year. One promising area of research is the use of CRISPR gene editing technology to specifically target and correct genetic mutations that cause leukemia. While this technology is still in the early stages of development, it has the potential to revolutionize leukemia treatment and lead to more personalized, effective therapies.

the advancements in leukemia research have led to improved treatment options and increased survival rates for patients. Targeted therapies, immunotherapy, and personalized treatment options based on genetic profiling are just a few examples of the progress being made. However, there is still much to be learned about leukemia and its treatment, and ongoing research is crucial in the fight against this disease. With continued efforts and funding, the hope is that one day we will find a cure for leukemia and other types of cancer.

Emerging Treatments

Leukemia is a type of cancer that affects the blood and bone marrow, and while there are many effective treatments available, there is still a need for better therapies. Emerging treatments offer hope for patients with leukemia, as these new therapies can improve outcomes and quality of life. In this essay, we will explore some of the latest emerging treatments for leukemia.

One emerging treatment for leukemia is chimeric antigen receptor (CAR) T-cell therapy. This treatment involves taking a patient's T cells and modifying them in a laboratory to recognize and attack leukemia cells. The modified T cells are then infused back into the patient's body. CAR T-cell therapy has shown promising results in clinical trials for patients with certain types of leukemia, including acute lymphoblastic leukemia (ALL) and chronic lymphocytic leukemia (CLL). In fact, in 2017, the FDA approved the first CAR T-cell therapy for the treatment of children and young adults with relapsed or refractory ALL.

Another emerging treatment for leukemia is targeted therapy. Targeted therapy involves using drugs that specifically target the genetic mutations that drive the growth of leukemia cells. These drugs are designed to interfere with specific molecules that are involved in the growth and division of cancer cells. Targeted therapies have shown significant benefits for patients with certain types of leukemia, including chronic myeloid leukemia (CML) and acute myeloid leukemia (AML). For example, drugs that target the BCR-ABL gene, which is involved in the development of CML, have revolutionized the treatment of this disease.

Immunotherapy is another emerging treatment for leukemia. Immunotherapy involves using the body's immune system to fight cancer cells. One type of immunotherapy that has shown promise in leukemia treatment is checkpoint inhibitors. Checkpoint inhibitors are drugs that block the immune system from being turned off by cancer cells. By blocking these signals, the immune system is better able to recognize and attack cancer cells. Clinical trials have shown promising results for checkpoint inhibitors in the treatment of CLL and AML.

Gene therapy is also an emerging treatment for leukemia. This therapy involves altering a patient's genes to treat or prevent disease. One type of gene therapy that has shown promise in leukemia treatment is called gene editing. Gene editing involves using molecular tools to edit a patient's genes in a precise way. This technique has been used in clinical trials to modify immune cells to attack leukemia cells more effectively.

In addition to these emerging treatments, there is ongoing research in other areas, such as epigenetic therapy, which involves modifying the activity of genes that contribute to cancer growth, and stem cell transplantation, which involves replacing damaged or diseased bone marrow with healthy stem cells. These and other emerging treatments offer hope for patients with leukemia and may lead to new and better therapies in the future.

While these emerging treatments show promise, it is important to note that they are still in the early stages of development and may not be widely available for some time. It is also important to note that not all patients will be eligible for these treatments, and that they may not be effective for everyone. Patients with leukemia should discuss all available treatment options with their healthcare provider to determine the best course of action.

emerging treatments offer hope for patients with leukemia. CAR T-cell therapy, targeted therapy, immunotherapy, gene therapy, and other emerging treatments have shown promise in clinical trials and may lead to better outcomes and quality of life for patients with leukemia. Ongoing research in these and other areas is essential for developing new and better therapies for this devastating disease.

Personalized Medicine and Precision Oncology

Personalized medicine and precision oncology are emerging fields of cancer treatment that hold great promise in the fight against leukemia. These approaches seek to tailor treatment to the individual patient based on the specific genetic and molecular characteristics of their cancer, with the goal of increasing treatment efficacy and minimizing side effects.

In traditional cancer treatment, patients are treated based on the type and stage of cancer they have. However, recent advances in technology have allowed researchers to better understand the genetic and molecular underpinnings of cancer. This has led to the development of new approaches to treatment that are more targeted and individualized.

One of the key tools used in personalized medicine and precision oncology is genomic sequencing. This technology allows researchers to analyze the DNA of cancer cells and identify specific genetic mutations or alterations that arc driving the growth and spread of the cancer. This information can then be used to develop targeted therapies that specifically target these mutations, while sparing healthy cells.

In leukemia, there are a number of specific genetic mutations that have been identified as driving the development and progression of the disease. For example, the BCR-ABL fusion gene is found in nearly all cases of chronic myeloid leukemia (CML), and is a major target for targeted therapies such as imatinib. Similarly, mutations in genes such as FLT3 and IDH1/2 are common in acute myeloid leukemia (AML) and are also the target of new therapies.

Another tool used in personalized medicine is the use of biomarkers to identify patients who are likely to respond to a particular therapy. For example, researchers have identified a biomarker known as PD-L1 that is associated with a response to immune checkpoint inhibitors, a type of immunotherapy. By identifying patients with high levels of PD-L1, doctors can select patients who are most likely to benefit from this type of therapy.

Precision oncology also involves the use of sophisticated computer algorithms to analyze large amounts of data and develop treatment recommendations. These algorithms take into account not only the patient's cancer type and stage, but also their genetic and molecular profile, as well as other factors such as their overall health and medical history.

One major advantage of personalized medicine and precision oncology is that it can potentially reduce the need for traditional chemotherapy, which can cause a range of side effects such as nausea, hair loss, and fatigue. By specifically targeting the cancer cells, these approaches can minimize damage to healthy cells and reduce the risk of side effects.

Another advantage is that personalized medicine can potentially improve the effectiveness of treatment. By targeting the specific genetic and molecular characteristics of the cancer, doctors can develop treatments that are more likely to be effective in individual patients.

Despite these promising advantages, there are still challenges to implementing personalized medicine and precision oncology in the clinic. One major challenge is the cost and availability of genetic testing and sequencing. These tests can be expensive and may not be covered by insurance, making them difficult for some patients to access.

There is also a need for more research to identify new genetic and molecular targets for treatment, as well as to validate the effectiveness of these approaches in clinical trials. As with any new treatment approach, it will be important to carefully evaluate the safety and efficacy of personalized medicine and precision oncology before they are widely adopted in clinical practice.

personalized medicine and precision oncology hold great promise in the treatment of leukemia and other cancers. By tailoring treatment to the individual patient based on their genetic and molecular profile, doctors can potentially improve treatment efficacy while minimizing side effects. While there are still challenges to implementing these approaches in the clinic, continued research and development in this field is likely to lead to new and more effective treatments for leukemia and other cancers in the future.

Chapter Seven

Coping with Leukemia

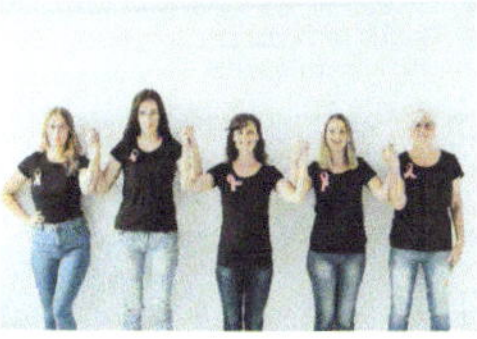

Coping with Leukemia can be challenging, both physically and emotionally. The diagnosis of Leukemia can be overwhelming and can have a significant impact on your life and your loved ones. However, there are many things you can do to help you cope and manage the effects of Leukemia.

1. Educate yourself: Learn as much as you can about Leukemia. Knowledge can help you better understand the disease and its treatment options, and help you feel more in control.

2. Stay connected: Build a support system of family, friends, and healthcare professionals who can offer you emotional support and practical help when you need it.

3. Take care of your physical health: Eat a healthy, well-balanced diet and get regular exercise. Rest when you need to and avoid exposure to infection.

4. Manage stress: Stress can make your symptoms worse and impact your overall health. Find ways to manage stress that work for you, such as meditation, yoga, or talking with a therapist.

5. Be open about your feelings: It is normal to experience a range of emotions when dealing with Leukemia, including fear, anxiety, sadness, and anger. Don't be afraid to express these feelings to loved ones or a mental health professional.

6. Seek out support groups: Joining a support group can provide you with an opportunity to connect with others who are going through similar experiences and share advice and encouragement.

7. Engage in activities that bring you joy: Participating in activities you enjoy, such as hobbies, spending time with loved ones, or volunteering, can help improve your overall mood and give you a sense of purpose.

Coping with Leukemia is a process that takes time and effort, but with the right support and resources, it is possible to live a fulfilling life with the disease.

Emotional impact of

Leukemia

Leukemia can have a significant emotional impact on both patients and their loved ones. A cancer diagnosis can be overwhelming, and it can be difficult to process the range of emotions that come with it. Common feelings include anxiety, depression, fear, and uncertainty.

Patients may also experience a sense of loss of control over their lives, as they may have to put their plans and goals on hold to focus on their treatment. The physical symptoms of Leukemia and its treatment can also affect a patient's emotional well-being, leading to fatigue, pain, and other symptoms.

For loved ones, watching someone they care about go through Leukemia can also be challenging. It's important to provide support and be there for the patient, but caregivers may also experience stress, anxiety, and a sense of helplessness.

Seeking support from friends, family, and healthcare professionals can help manage these emotions. Counseling and therapy can also be beneficial in providing an outlet for patients and caregivers to express their feelings and concerns.

It's important to remember that it's normal to experience a range of emotions during a Leukemia diagnosis and treatment. It's okay to seek help and support, and with time and appropriate care, patients and their loved ones can learn to cope with the emotional impact of Leukemia.

Coping strategies for patients and caregivers

Coping with Leukemia can be overwhelming for both the patient and the caregiver. It is essential to have a good support system and to take care of yourself to manage the stress and emotions that come with the diagnosis and treatment. Here are some coping strategies for patients and caregivers:

Educate yourself: Learn as much as you can about the disease, the treatment options, and potential side effects. This will help you feel more in control of the situation and make informed decisions.

Build a support network: Connect with family, friends, and support groups to share your feelings and experiences. This can help you feel less isolated and provide emotional support.

Stay active: Exercise can help reduce stress and anxiety, boost your mood, and improve overall well-being. It can also help combat the side effects of treatment.

Take care of yourself: Eat a healthy, balanced diet, get enough rest, and avoid alcohol and smoking. Take time for activities you enjoy and practice relaxation techniques, such as meditation or yoga.

Communicate with your healthcare team: Keep an open dialogue with your doctor and other members of your healthcare team. Discuss any concerns you have and ask questions about your treatment plan.

Consider therapy: Counseling or therapy can be helpful in managing the emotional impact of Leukemia. It can provide a safe space to express your feelings and learn coping skills.

Find joy in the small things: Focus on the positive and find joy in the small things in life. This can help improve your mood and provide a sense of happiness and fulfillment.

Remember, coping with Leukemia is a process, and it is normal to have good days and bad days. Be patient with yourself and take it one day at a time. With the right support, self-care, and coping strategies, it is possible to manage the emotional impact of Leukemia and improve quality of life.

Emotional and Psychological Support

Emotional and psychological support is an essential aspect of the care for individuals with leukemia. The diagnosis and treatment of leukemia can be a challenging and stressful experience, and patients and their families may experience a range of emotions, including fear, anxiety, depression, and frustration. Emotional and psychological support can help patients cope with their diagnosis, manage their symptoms, and improve their overall quality of life.

Leukemia is a type of cancer that affects the blood and bone marrow. It is a chronic condition that requires ongoing treatment, including chemotherapy, radiation therapy, and stem cell transplantation. The physical symptoms of leukemia, such as fatigue, fever, and pain, can be debilitating and can impact a patient's quality of life. However, the emotional and psychological effects of leukemia are also significant and cannot be overlooked.

One of the most important aspects of emotional and psychological support for patients with leukemia is communication. Patients and their families need to feel comfortable communicating with their healthcare team about their concerns, fears, and questions. Open and honest communication can help patients better understand their diagnosis, treatment options, and potential side effects. It can also help patients feel more in control of their care and decision-making.

In addition to communication, patients with leukemia may benefit from counseling and psychotherapy. Counseling can help patients cope with the emotional and psychological effects of their diagnosis and treatment. It can also provide patients with practical strategies for managing stress, anxiety, and depression. Psychotherapy, such as cognitive-behavioral therapy (CBT), can help patients identify negative thought patterns and behaviors and replace them with more positive and adaptive ones.

Support groups can also be an excellent source of emotional and psychological support for patients with leukemia. Support groups can provide patients with a sense of community and shared experience. Patients can share their experiences, concerns, and coping strategies with others who understand what they are going through. Support groups can also provide patients with practical information about managing their symptoms and improving their overall quality of life.

Family members of patients with leukemia may also require emotional and psychological support. The diagnosis and treatment of leukemia can be a challenging and stressful experience for family members, who may feel overwhelmed, anxious, or depressed. Family members may also need support in managing the practical aspects of caring for a loved one with leukemia, such as administering medications and managing appointments.

Emotional and psychological support for patients with leukemia is not a one-size-fits-all approach. Patients have unique needs and preferences, and their emotional and psychological support should be tailored to meet their individual needs. Healthcare providers should take a patient-centered approach to emotional and psychological support, working closely with patients and their families to understand their needs and preferences.

emotional and psychological support is an essential aspect of the care for individuals with leukemia. The diagnosis and treatment of leukemia can be a challenging and stressful experience, and patients and their families may experience a range of emotions. Effective emotional and psychological support can help patients cope with their diagnosis, manage their symptoms, and improve their overall quality of life. Communication, counseling and psychotherapy, support groups, and tailored patient-centered care are all important components of emotional and psychological support for patients with leukemia.

Pain Management

Leukemia is a type of cancer that affects the blood and bone marrow, and it can cause pain in different parts of the body. Pain management is an essential aspect of leukemia treatment, as it can significantly improve the patient's quality of life.

The pain in leukemia can be caused by various factors, including the disease itself, chemotherapy, radiation therapy, and complications such as infections or bleeding. The type, severity, and location of pain can vary depending on the stage of the disease and the patient's overall health. Common sites of pain include the bones, joints, and abdomen.

One of the primary goals of pain management in leukemia is to control the pain effectively while minimizing the side effects of pain medications. The management approach depends on the patient's individual needs and may involve several different methods, including medication, non-pharmacological interventions, and complementary therapies.

Pain medications are typically the first line of treatment for leukemia-related pain. Analgesics, such as non-steroidal anti-inflammatory drugs (NSAIDs) and opioids, are commonly used to manage mild to moderate pain. However, opioids may have side effects, such as nausea, constipation, and sedation, and they can also be habit-forming. Thus, they are typically reserved for severe pain or for short-term use. In some cases, other medications, such as antidepressants or anticonvulsants, may be prescribed to treat neuropathic pain or other specific types of pain.

Non-pharmacological interventions can also be effective in managing leukemia-related pain. These may include physical therapy, exercise, massage, and acupuncture. Physical therapy and exercise can help improve mobility and reduce pain by strengthening the muscles and joints. Massage and acupuncture can help reduce tension and promote relaxation, which can help alleviate pain.

Complementary therapies, such as aromatherapy and meditation, may also be useful in managing leukemia-related pain. Aromatherapy involves the use of essential oils, which can be inhaled or applied topically to help reduce pain and promote relaxation. Meditation and other mind-body techniques can also help reduce stress and anxiety, which can contribute to pain.

In addition to managing pain, supportive care is also essential in leukemia treatment. This includes managing symptoms, such as nausea and fatigue, as well as preventing and treating infections. Patients with leukemia are at increased risk of infections due to the weakened immune system, so it is crucial to take steps to prevent infections, such as hand hygiene, vaccination, and avoiding contact with sick individuals.

In summary, pain management is an essential aspect of leukemia treatment, and a multidisciplinary approach may be necessary to effectively manage pain and other symptoms. Pain medications, non-pharmacological interventions, and complementary therapies can all be effective in managing leukemia-related pain. Additionally, supportive care is critical in leukemia treatment, including infection prevention and management, and addressing other symptoms that may contribute to pain. By effectively managing pain and providing comprehensive supportive care, patients with leukemia can improve their quality of life and overall outcomes.

The role of diet in

Leukemia

The role of diet in the treatment of Leukemia is an area of ongoing research. While a specific diet has not been shown to cure Leukemia, eating a well-balanced diet can help patients maintain their strength and energy during treatment.

One of the main concerns for Leukemia patients is maintaining a healthy immune system. This can be accomplished through consuming foods that are high in vitamins and minerals, such as fruits and vegetables. A diet that includes a variety of colorful fruits and vegetables can help ensure that patients are getting the nutrients they need to stay healthy.

Another important consideration is maintaining a healthy weight. Patients with Leukemia may experience weight loss due to the disease or the side effects of treatment. Eating a healthy, balanced diet can help patients maintain their weight and avoid malnutrition.

Some patients may also experience mouth sores, nausea, or difficulty swallowing during treatment. In these cases, a soft food or liquid diet may be recommended. Patients should work with their healthcare team to develop a nutrition plan that meets their individual needs.

It's important to note that some dietary supplements and herbal remedies may interact with cancer treatments or cause harmful side effects. Patients should always consult with their healthcare team before taking any supplements or herbal remedies.

In summary, a well-balanced diet can help Leukemia patients maintain their strength and energy during treatment, support a healthy immune system, and avoid malnutrition. Patients should work with their healthcare team to develop a nutrition plan that meets their individual needs.

The role of stress in

Leukemia

There is no clear evidence that stress causes Leukemia or worsens its outcome, but managing stress is still important for overall well-being and quality of life for both patients and caregivers. Leukemia can be a stressful and overwhelming diagnosis, and coping with treatment and potential complications can add to this stress.

It is important to develop healthy coping mechanisms to manage stress, such as exercise, meditation, yoga, or other activities that you enjoy. Joining a support group for patients and caregivers can also provide a valuable outlet for sharing experiences and connecting with others who are going through similar situations.

In addition, it is important to communicate openly with healthcare providers about any concerns or stressors you may be experiencing. They may be able to provide additional resources or support to help you manage stress and improve your overall well-being.

What are the risks and complications associated with

Leukemia

?

Leukemia can cause several complications that can be life-threatening. Some of the risks and complications associated with Leukemia include:

Infections: Leukemia can weaken the immune system, making the body more vulnerable to infections.

Bleeding and clotting: Leukemia can affect the normal clotting process, leading to bleeding or clotting problems.

Anemia: Leukemia can cause a decrease in the number of red blood cells in the body, leading to anemia.

Organ damage: Leukemia cells can accumulate in different organs and tissues, causing damage to them. This can result in problems such as liver or kidney failure.

Recurrence: Even after successful treatment, Leukemia can sometimes recur, requiring additional treatment.

Side effects of treatment: Treatment for Leukemia can have several side effects, such as nausea, vomiting, fatigue, and hair loss.

Secondary cancers: Some of the treatments for Leukemia, such as chemotherapy and radiation, can increase the risk of developing secondary cancers later in life.

It is important for patients to work closely with their healthcare providers to manage and monitor these risks and complications. With proper care and management, many patients are able to successfully manage their Leukemia and lead fulfilling lives.

Chapter Eight

Living with Leukemia

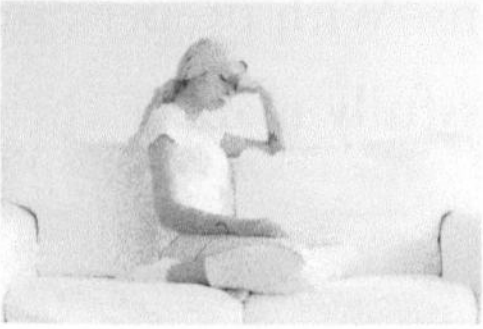

Leukemia is a life-changing diagnosis that can be difficult to come to terms with. Living with Leukemia requires a strong support system, as well as a willingness to adapt to a new way of life.

One of the most important things for Leukemia patients is to communicate with their healthcare team. This means keeping appointments, asking questions, and reporting any new symptoms or concerns. It's also important to keep track of medications and side effects, and to make adjustments as needed.

In addition to medical care, emotional support is also crucial for those living with Leukemia. Support groups can provide an opportunity to connect with others who are going through similar experiences, as well as a space to share feelings and challenges. Family and friends can also play a role in providing emotional support, and may be able to help with day-to-day tasks.

Maintaining a healthy lifestyle is also important for Leukemia patients. This can include following a balanced diet, getting regular exercise, and getting enough sleep. It's also important to avoid smoking and limit alcohol consumption, as these can have a negative impact on overall health.

Finally, it's important for those living with Leukemia to take care of their mental health. This can include seeking professional help if needed, practicing stress-reducing techniques such as meditation or yoga, and finding activities that bring joy and fulfillment.

Living with Leukemia can be challenging, but with the right support, resources, and mindset, it's possible to lead a fulfilling life.

Palliative Care and Hospice

Leukemia is a serious illness that requires complex medical treatments, often causing significant physical, emotional, and psychological strain on the patient and their loved ones. In some cases, despite the best efforts of medical professionals, leukemia may be terminal, and patients may require palliative care and hospice services. Palliative care and hospice focus on the comfort and quality of life for patients facing life-threatening illnesses. This essay will discuss the importance of palliative care and hospice in leukemia treatment, the differences between these two types of care, and the benefits they provide.

Palliative care is specialized medical care designed to provide relief from the symptoms and stress of serious illnesses like leukemia. Its goal is to improve the quality of life for both the patient and their family. Palliative care is available at any stage of the disease, regardless of the patient's age or the extent of their illness. It is not the same as hospice care, which is a specialized form of palliative care designed for those who have been given six months or less to live.

The palliative care team is made up of doctors, nurses, social workers, and other healthcare professionals who work together to manage the patient's symptoms, such as pain, fatigue, and nausea, among others. They also offer emotional and psychological support to patients and their families, helping them to cope with the stress and anxiety associated with the illness.

One of the benefits of palliative care is that it can be provided alongside curative treatments, such as chemotherapy or radiation therapy. Palliative care can help to manage the side effects of these treatments, such as fatigue or pain, which can improve the patient's quality of life. It can also help patients make informed decisions about their care, based on their individual needs and goals.

Hospice care, on the other hand, is specialized care designed for those who are nearing the end of their life, and who have decided to stop pursuing curative treatments. Hospice care can be provided at home, in a hospice facility, or in a hospital, and is focused on providing comfort and support to patients and their families.

The hospice care team is also made up of doctors, nurses, social workers, and other healthcare professionals who provide care and support to patients and their families. Hospice care can provide a range of services, including pain management, emotional and spiritual support, and counseling. It can also help patients and their families make end-of-life decisions and plan for the future.

One of the benefits of hospice care is that it can provide patients with a peaceful and comfortable end of life experience. It can also help families to cope with the emotional and practical challenges that come with caring for a loved one who is dying. Hospice care can also help to ensure that the patient's wishes are respected, and that they are able to pass away with dignity.

palliative care and hospice are important aspects of leukemia treatment, providing patients with relief from symptoms, emotional and psychological support, and comfort during the end-of-life journey. Palliative care can be provided at any stage of the disease and can be provided alongside curative treatments, whereas hospice care is designed for those who have decided to stop pursuing curative treatments and are nearing the end of their life. Both forms of care can help patients and their families cope with the physical, emotional, and psychological challenges associated with leukemia, and can ensure that the patient is able to pass away with dignity and respect.

Goals of Palliative Care

Palliative care is a specialized medical care that aims to improve the quality of life of patients and their families facing life-threatening illnesses, including leukemia. The goal of palliative care is to prevent or treat symptoms and side effects, manage pain, and provide emotional and spiritual support. Palliative care is not limited to end-of-life care but can be provided to patients at any stage of their illness. In this essay, we will discuss the goals of palliative care for leukemia patients.

One of the primary goals of palliative care for leukemia patients is to alleviate symptoms and side effects associated with the disease and its treatment. Leukemia treatment, such as chemotherapy and radiation, can cause several side effects, such as nausea, vomiting, fatigue, and pain. Palliative care can provide medications, therapies, and other interventions to help manage these symptoms and improve the patient's quality of life. By reducing the burden of symptoms and side effects, palliative care can help patients continue their treatment and improve their overall well-being.

Another essential goal of palliative care for leukemia patients is to improve their emotional and psychological well-being. Patients with leukemia can experience a range of emotional and psychological issues, such as anxiety, depression, and fear. Palliative care can provide emotional and spiritual support to help patients cope with the emotional impact of their illness.

This support can come in the form of counseling, support groups, and spiritual care. By addressing the emotional and psychological needs of patients, palliative care can help them feel more in control and improve their overall quality of life.

Palliative care can also provide support for the families and caregivers of leukemia patients. Caring for a loved one with leukemia can be challenging and emotionally exhausting. Palliative care can offer family counseling and support groups to help caregivers cope with their own emotional and psychological needs. Palliative care can also help families navigate the complexities of the healthcare system and make informed decisions about the care of their loved ones.

For patients with advanced leukemia, the goals of palliative care may shift towards end-of-life care. In these cases, the primary goal of palliative care is to provide comfort and support to the patient and their family. This may involve managing symptoms, providing spiritual and emotional support, and helping the patient and their family prepare for the end of life. Palliative care can also assist with advance care planning, such as determining the patient's goals of care and preferences for end-of-life care.

the goals of palliative care for leukemia patients are centered around improving the quality of life of patients and their families facing life-threatening illnesses. Palliative care can help manage symptoms and side effects, provide emotional and psychological support, and assist with end-of-life care. By addressing the needs of patients and their families, palliative care can help them cope with the challenges of leukemia and improve their overall well-being.

Managing Symptoms

Leukemia is a type of cancer that affects the blood and bone marrow, and it can cause a variety of symptoms that may affect a patient's quality of life. While treatments such as chemotherapy, radiation, and stem cell transplants can help to manage the cancer itself, managing symptoms through palliative care is also an important part of leukemia treatment. Palliative care is an approach to care that aims to improve the quality of life of patients and their families who are facing life-threatening illnesses.

Managing symptoms of leukemia can be a challenging process, as different patients may experience different symptoms at varying levels of severity. Some common symptoms of leukemia include fatigue, fever, bone pain, bleeding or bruising easily, infections, weight loss, and difficulty breathing. Palliative care can help manage these symptoms by providing relief through medications, counseling, and other supportive services.

One of the most common symptoms of leukemia is fatigue, which can be caused by the cancer itself, chemotherapy, or other treatments. Palliative care can help manage fatigue through energy conservation techniques, such as scheduling rest periods throughout the day, and by providing support for physical activity and exercise. Patients can also benefit from counseling and support groups to help manage the emotional toll of fatigue and cancer treatment.

Fever is another common symptom of leukemia, and it can be caused by infection or the cancer itself. Palliative care can help manage fever through medications such as acetaminophen or ibuprofen, as well as by providing support for hydration and rest. In addition, supportive care services such as nutritional counseling and physical therapy can help to manage fever by promoting overall health and wellness.

Bone pain is another common symptom of leukemia, and it can be caused by the cancer spreading to the bones or by treatments such as chemotherapy. Palliative care can help manage bone pain through medications such as opioids, as well as through physical therapy and other supportive services. In addition, counseling and support groups can help patients manage the emotional toll of chronic pain and cancer treatment.

Bleeding or bruising easily is another common symptom of leukemia, and it can be caused by the cancer itself or by treatments such as chemotherapy. Palliative care can help manage bleeding and bruising through medications such as platelet transfusions or clotting factor replacement, as well as through counseling and support services to manage the emotional toll of living with a bleeding disorder.

Infections are a common complication of leukemia and can be caused by the cancer itself or by treatments such as chemotherapy. Palliative care can help manage infections through antibiotics, antiviral medications, and other supportive services such as nutritional counseling and physical therapy. In addition, counseling and support groups can help patients manage the emotional toll of living with an infection and cancer treatment.

Weight loss is another common symptom of leukemia, and it can be caused by the cancer itself or by treatments such as chemotherapy. Palliative care can help manage weight loss through nutritional counseling and support, as well as by providing medications to increase appetite and manage nausea and vomiting. Counseling and support groups can also help patients manage the emotional toll of living with a chronic illness and the impact it can have on their body image and self-esteem.

Difficulty breathing is a less common symptom of leukemia, but it can occur if the cancer affects the lungs or if treatments such as chemotherapy or radiation cause lung damage. Palliative care can help manage difficulty breathing through medications such as bronchodilators, as well as through counseling and support services to manage anxiety and other emotional responses to breathing difficulties.

Hospice Care

Hospice care is a form of medical care that is provided to patients with life-limiting illnesses, with the aim of providing comfort and support to both the patient and their family. Hospice care is typically initiated when a patient has a terminal diagnosis, and further curative treatment is no longer possible or desired. Hospice care is designed to provide a peaceful and comfortable end-of-life experience for the patient, while also addressing the emotional and spiritual needs of the patient and their family.

Leukemia is a type of cancer that affects the blood and bone marrow, and it is a disease that can progress quickly and aggressively. As with other types of cancer, leukemia can be challenging to manage and can require intensive treatment such as chemotherapy, radiation therapy, and stem cell transplantation. However, in some cases, these treatments may not be effective, and the disease may progress to the point where further treatment is no longer possible or desirable.

When a patient with leukemia is no longer a candidate for curative treatment, hospice care may be a viable option. Hospice care can provide a range of services to patients with leukemia, including pain management, symptom relief, emotional support, and spiritual care. The goals of hospice care are to improve the quality of life for patients and their families, while also helping to maintain their dignity and sense of control.

One of the primary benefits of hospice care for patients with leukemia is pain management. Leukemia can cause significant pain, including bone pain, headaches, and abdominal pain. Hospice care teams are trained to manage these symptoms effectively, using a range of medications and other therapies to provide relief. Hospice teams can also provide emotional and psychological support to patients, helping them to cope with the physical and emotional challenges of their illness.

In addition to pain management, hospice care can also help manage other symptoms associated with leukemia, such as fatigue, nausea, and shortness of breath. Hospice care teams can provide a range of services to help patients manage these symptoms, including medications, oxygen therapy, and counseling.

Another benefit of hospice care for patients with leukemia is the emotional support that is available. The diagnosis of leukemia can be overwhelming for patients and their families, and hospice care teams can help patients and their families cope with the emotional challenges of the disease. Hospice care teams can provide counseling and support to patients and their families, helping them to address their fears and concerns about the disease and the end of life.

Finally, hospice care can provide spiritual support to patients and their families. Many patients with leukemia may have strong spiritual beliefs, and hospice care teams can work with patients to provide spiritual care that is aligned with their beliefs. This can include working with spiritual leaders or providing access to spiritual resources that can help patients and their families find comfort and peace.

Survivorship

Survivorship is an important concept in the treatment of leukemia, as more and more people are living longer after a diagnosis of this disease. Survivorship refers to the process of living with and beyond cancer, including the physical, emotional, and social aspects of recovery. Survivors of leukemia face unique challenges, such as the long-term effects of treatment, the risk of relapse, and the need for ongoing monitoring and support. This essay will explore the concept of survivorship in the context of leukemia, including the challenges that survivors face, strategies for coping and adjusting to life after cancer, and the importance of ongoing care and support.

One of the most significant challenges facing leukemia survivors is the long-term effects of treatment. Chemotherapy, radiation, and other treatments used to treat leukemia can cause a variety of side effects, including fatigue, pain, cognitive impairment, and emotional distress. These effects may persist long after treatment has ended, and can significantly impact survivors' quality of life. For example, some survivors may experience peripheral neuropathy, a condition characterized by numbness, tingling, and pain in the hands and feet. Others may experience cognitive problems such as memory loss, difficulty concentrating, and mental fog. These long-term effects can be particularly challenging for survivors who are trying to return to work or school, as they can impact their ability to perform everyday tasks.

Another challenge facing leukemia survivors is the risk of relapse. While many people are cured of leukemia, some survivors may experience a recurrence of the disease. This can be a frightening and stressful experience, and may require additional treatment such as chemotherapy or stem cell transplant. Survivors may also experience anxiety and fear about the possibility of relapse, which can impact their emotional well-being and quality of life. For this reason, ongoing monitoring and surveillance is important for survivors of leukemia, as it can help detect any signs of relapse early and ensure that appropriate treatment is provided.

Coping with the emotional and psychological impact of cancer is another important aspect of survivorship. Many survivors of leukemia experience a range of emotions, including anxiety, depression, and fear. These feelings may be related to the trauma of the cancer diagnosis, the stress of treatment, or the uncertainty of the future. Coping with these emotions can be challenging, but there are strategies that survivors can use to help manage their feelings. For example, talking to a counselor or therapist can be helpful, as can joining a support group or engaging in mindfulness-based practices like meditation and yoga.

Physical activity and exercise are also important components of survivorship. Exercise has been shown to improve physical and emotional health, reduce the risk of recurrence, and improve quality of life for cancer survivors. Survivors of leukemia may need to adjust their exercise routines to account for any physical limitations or side effects of treatment. However, even gentle forms of exercise like walking or swimming can provide important benefits for survivors.

Finally, ongoing care and support is critical for survivors of leukemia. Survivors may need ongoing monitoring to detect any signs of relapse or long-term effects of treatment. They may also need support to manage the emotional and psychological challenges of survivorship. This may include regular check-ups with a healthcare provider, access to counseling or therapy, and participation in survivorship programs or support groups. Family and friends can also play an important role in supporting survivors, by providing emotional support, helping with everyday tasks, and participating in survivorship activities.

survivorship is an important aspect of leukemia treatment, as more and more people are living longer after a diagnosis of this disease. Survivors of leukemia face unique challenges, including the long-term effects of treatment, the risk of relapse, and the emotional impact of cancer. However, there are strategies that survivors can use to manage these challenges, including physical activity, counseling, and ongoing care and support.

Follow-Up Care

Follow-up care is a critical aspect of managing and treating leukemia. After initial treatment, patients must continue to undergo regular check-ups and follow-up care to ensure that the disease does not recur, and to manage any long-term effects of treatment. In this essay, we will discuss the importance of follow-up care for leukemia patients and the various aspects of care that are involved.

The goal of follow-up care is to monitor the patient's health, detect any signs of recurrence, manage long-term side effects of treatment, and provide emotional support. Follow-up care is typically managed by a team of healthcare professionals, including the patient's primary care physician, oncologist, and other specialists as needed. The frequency and duration of follow-up care depend on various factors, such as the patient's age, stage of leukemia, type of treatment, and overall health.

One of the most critical aspects of follow-up care is monitoring the patient's blood cell counts. Blood tests are essential to detect any abnormalities and determine if leukemia cells are present. Patients who have undergone bone marrow or stem cell transplants may require more frequent blood tests. Additionally, monitoring for any new or recurring symptoms is also important. These may include fatigue, fever, unexplained weight loss, or other symptoms that may indicate a recurrence of leukemia.

Another critical aspect of follow-up care is managing long-term side effects of treatment. Chemotherapy and radiation therapy can cause a range of side effects, such as fatigue, nausea, and hair loss. These side effects can last for several months or even years after treatment. Patients may require ongoing medical care to manage these symptoms and prevent them from interfering with their daily lives.

Patients may also require emotional and psychological support after treatment. Many leukemia patients experience anxiety, depression, and other emotional disturbances. These issues can be addressed through counseling or other support services, such as support groups, which can help patients cope with the emotional and psychological challenges of cancer survivorship.

Additionally, patients may require ongoing nutritional support and physical therapy. Leukemia and its treatments can affect a patient's appetite, making it difficult for them to get the nutrients they need to stay healthy. Physical therapy can help patients regain strength and flexibility after treatment and improve their overall quality of life.

Follow-up care may also involve managing the patient's medications. Patients who are taking medications to manage their leukemia may require ongoing monitoring to ensure that the drugs are working effectively and to prevent any adverse reactions.

Finally, follow-up care may involve regular cancer screenings to detect any new or recurring cancers. Patients who have had leukemia are at a higher risk of developing other cancers, so regular screenings are essential to detect any potential issues early.

follow-up care is a critical aspect of managing and treating leukemia. It involves monitoring the patient's health, detecting any signs of recurrence, managing long-term side effects of treatment, providing emotional support, and addressing any other issues that may arise. The goal of follow-up care is to ensure that leukemia patients continue to receive the care and support they need to live healthy, fulfilling lives after treatment. By working with a team of healthcare professionals, leukemia patients can receive comprehensive, individualized follow-up care that meets their unique needs and helps them achieve the best possible outcomes.

Late Effects and Secondary Cancers

Leukemia is a type of cancer that affects the blood and bone marrow, and it can require intensive treatments such as chemotherapy, radiation, and stem cell transplantation. While these treatments can be successful in fighting the cancer, they can also have long-term effects on the body. In this essay, we will explore the late effects and secondary cancers associated with leukemia treatments, and how follow-up care can help mitigate these risks.

Late effects refer to the health problems that can occur months or even years after cancer treatment has ended. These late effects can be caused by a number of factors, including the cancer itself, the treatments used to fight it, and the patient's individual health history. Some common late effects of leukemia treatments include:

1. Reduced fertility: Chemotherapy and radiation can damage the ovaries or testes, leading to reduced fertility or infertility.

2. Growth problems: Children who undergo leukemia treatment may experience delays in growth and development.

3. Neurocognitive problems: Chemotherapy and radiation can damage the brain, leading to problems with memory, attention, and learning.

4. Cardiovascular problems: Certain chemotherapy drugs can damage the heart and blood vessels, increasing the risk of heart disease.

5. Thyroid problems: Radiation to the neck area can damage the thyroid gland, leading to thyroid problems.

In addition to these late effects, leukemia survivors also have an increased risk of developing secondary cancers. This is because the treatments used to fight leukemia can damage healthy cells, leading to genetic mutations that can cause new cancers to form. The risk of secondary cancers varies depending on the type of treatment and the patient's individual health history, but some common secondary cancers associated with leukemia treatments include:

6. Acute myeloid leukemia (AML): Patients who undergo chemotherapy and radiation for leukemia have an increased risk of developing AML, which is a type of blood cancer.

7. Solid tumors: Radiation therapy can increase the risk of developing solid tumors such as breast cancer or lung cancer.

While these late effects and secondary cancers can be concerning, it's important to remember that not all leukemia survivors will experience them. Many factors can influence a patient's risk, including the type and duration of treatment, the patient's age and health history, and lifestyle factors such as smoking and exercise.

To help mitigate these risks, it's important for leukemia survivors to receive appropriate follow-up care. This care can include regular physical exams, blood tests, and imaging scans to monitor for late effects and secondary cancers. In addition, survivors may benefit from working with a team of healthcare professionals, including oncologists, primary care doctors, and specialists such as cardiologists and endocrinologists.

Lifestyle factors can also play a role in reducing the risk of late effects and secondary cancers. For example, survivors can reduce their risk of heart disease by maintaining a healthy weight, eating a balanced diet, and getting regular exercise. They can also reduce their risk of secondary cancers by avoiding tobacco and limiting their exposure to other cancer-causing substances such as ultraviolet radiation.

In addition to physical health concerns, survivors may also experience emotional and psychological challenges. The experience of cancer and its treatments can be traumatic, and survivors may experience anxiety, depression, or post-traumatic stress disorder (PTSD). It's important for survivors to receive appropriate emotional support, which can include therapy, support groups, and other resources.

while leukemia treatments can be successful in fighting the cancer, they can also have long-term effects on the body, including late effects and an increased risk of secondary cancers. It's important for survivors to receive appropriate follow-up care and to take steps to reduce their risk of these complications. With the right care and support, leukemia survivors can lead healthy, fulfilling lives after cancer.

Caregiving and Family Support

Caregiving and Family Support in the context of leukemia can be a challenging and emotional experience. Leukemia is a type of cancer that affects the blood and bone marrow, and it requires ongoing medical care and support. The disease not only affects the person diagnosed with leukemia but also their family members and caregivers.

Caregiving involves a range of responsibilities, including administering medications, managing symptoms, accompanying the patient to medical appointments, and providing emotional support. Family members often take on the role of caregiver, and the experience can be both rewarding and challenging.

One of the most important aspects of caregiving is ensuring that the patient receives the best medical care possible. This can involve researching treatment options, communicating with medical professionals, and advocating for the patient's needs. Caregivers can also assist with medication management, ensuring that the patient takes their medications as prescribed and monitoring for any potential side effects.

Leukemia can cause a range of physical and emotional symptoms, and caregivers can play a critical role in managing these symptoms. This can involve assisting with activities of daily living, such as bathing and dressing, and monitoring for changes in the patient's health. Caregivers can also provide emotional support, which can involve listening to the patient's concerns and providing comfort and reassurance.

In addition to providing care, caregivers also need support themselves. Caring for a loved one with leukemia can be emotionally and physically exhausting, and caregivers may experience feelings of stress, anxiety, and depression. It is important for caregivers to take care of their own health and well-being, which can involve seeking support from family and friends, attending support groups, and taking breaks when needed.

Family members can also provide valuable support for the patient, which can involve assisting with daily tasks, providing emotional support, and advocating for the patient's needs. Family members can also play a critical role in helping the patient adjust to life with leukemia, which can involve making lifestyle changes and coping with the emotional impact of the disease.

Communication is also an essential component of caregiving and family support. It is important for caregivers and family members to communicate openly and honestly with each other and with the patient. This can involve discussing treatment options, managing expectations, and providing emotional support.

Leukemia can be a challenging and emotional experience for both patients and their families. Caregiving and family support can play a critical role in helping the patient manage their symptoms, navigate medical care, and cope with the emotional impact of the disease. By working together, caregivers and family members can provide valuable support and ensure that the patient receives the best possible care.

Roles and Responsibilities

Leukemia is a type of cancer that affects the blood and bone marrow, and it can be a very challenging disease to manage. Patients diagnosed with leukemia require comprehensive care that extends beyond medical treatment to ensure their physical and emotional needs are met. The care of a person with leukemia is often shared between healthcare professionals, caregivers, and family members. In this essay, we will discuss the roles and responsibilities of those involved in caring for someone with leukemia.

Healthcare Professionals

Healthcare professionals play a crucial role in the care of leukemia patients. They are responsible for diagnosing and treating the disease, monitoring symptoms, and managing side effects. They include hematologists, oncologists, nurses, pharmacists, and other specialists who work together to provide a comprehensive care plan for the patient.

Hematologists and oncologists are physicians who specialize in the treatment of blood cancers such as leukemia. They are responsible for determining the best treatment plan for the patient, which may include chemotherapy, radiation therapy, or stem cell transplant, among others. Nurses are also an integral part of the healthcare team, as they provide patient education, administer medication, and monitor the patient's vital signs.

Pharmacists play a vital role in the care of leukemia patients, as they are responsible for ensuring that medications are prescribed correctly and that the patient is taking them as prescribed. They also monitor for potential drug interactions and advise the healthcare team on the best medications to manage the patient's symptoms.

Caregivers

Caregivers play an essential role in caring for someone with leukemia. They are usually family members or close friends who provide physical and emotional support to the patient. Caregivers can assist with activities of daily living such as bathing, dressing, and meal preparation, as well as providing transportation to medical appointments.

Caregivers may also be responsible for managing the patient's medication regimen, monitoring symptoms, and communicating with the healthcare team. They must also be aware of potential side effects of treatment and know when to seek medical attention. Caregiving can be physically and emotionally demanding, and it is essential for caregivers to take care of themselves as well.

Family Members

Family members of leukemia patients also play a critical role in the care of their loved one. They can provide emotional support and help the patient maintain a positive outlook. Family members can also assist with caregiving duties, such as providing transportation to medical appointments or helping with household chores.

It is essential for family members to be informed about the patient's treatment plan and to be aware of potential side effects. They should also be prepared to offer assistance and support as needed. Communication is key in supporting a loved one with leukemia, and family members should be encouraged to ask questions and communicate their concerns to the healthcare team.

Patient

The patient is the most critical member of the care team, as they are the ones undergoing treatment and experiencing the effects of the disease. Patients with leukemia must take an active role in their care by following the treatment plan, reporting any symptoms or side effects, and communicating their concerns to the healthcare team.

Patients with leukemia may also benefit from support groups, counseling, and other resources to help them cope with the emotional and psychological effects of the disease. It is essential for patients to maintain a positive outlook and engage in activities that bring them joy and fulfillment.

caring for someone with leukemia requires a team approach that involves healthcare professionals, caregivers, family members, and the patient themselves. Each member of the care team has a specific role and responsibility in ensuring that the patient's physical and emotional needs are met. Effective communication and collaboration are essential to provide the best possible care for someone with leukemia.

Communication and Decision-Making

Communication and decision-making are essential components of the management of leukemia. The diagnosis of leukemia can be overwhelming and cause a great deal of stress for the patient and their loved ones. Effective communication between the healthcare team and the patient and their family is critical to ensuring that the patient receives the best possible care and treatment.

One of the most important aspects of communication is the ability to provide clear and concise information about the disease, its treatment options, and potential outcomes. Patients and their families need to understand the disease and its prognosis to make informed decisions about treatment options. The healthcare team must be sensitive to the emotional impact of the diagnosis and treatment and ensure that the patient and their family feel comfortable asking questions and expressing concerns.

The healthcare team must also be able to communicate effectively among themselves. Leukemia is often managed by a team of healthcare professionals, including hematologists, oncologists, radiation therapists, and other specialists. Effective communication among team members is critical to ensure that the patient receives the best possible care. The team must be able to share information about the patient's condition, discuss treatment options, and coordinate care.

In addition to effective communication, decision-making is also an important aspect of managing leukemia. Treatment decisions must be based on the patient's individual needs, preferences, and medical history. The healthcare team must work with the patient and their family to make decisions that are in the patient's best interest.

Treatment decisions for leukemia often involve a combination of chemotherapy, radiation therapy, and other supportive measures. The healthcare team must consider the potential benefits and risks of each treatment option and discuss these with the patient and their family. They must also take into account the patient's overall health, age, and other medical conditions when making treatment decisions.

Communication and decision-making also play an important role in managing the side effects of treatment. Many of the treatments for leukemia can cause side effects that can be difficult for patients to manage. The healthcare team must be able to provide information about these side effects and work with the patient and their family to develop strategies for managing them.

Supportive care is an essential part of managing leukemia, and effective communication and decision-making are critical to ensuring that the patient receives the best possible care. The healthcare team must be able to provide emotional support to the patient and their family throughout the course of treatment. They must also be able to provide information about resources that can help the patient and their family cope with the emotional and practical aspects of the disease.

effective communication and decision-making are essential components of managing leukemia. The healthcare team must be able to provide clear and concise information about the disease, its treatment options, and potential outcomes. They must also be able to communicate effectively among themselves to ensure that the patient receives the best possible care. Treatment decisions must be based on the patient's individual needs, preferences, and medical history. The healthcare team must work with the patient and their family to make decisions that are in the patient's best interest. Finally, the healthcare team must provide emotional support to the patient and their family throughout the course of treatment.

Resources for Caregivers

Leukemia is a type of cancer that affects the blood and bone marrow, which are responsible for producing blood cells. It can be a difficult diagnosis for patients, but it also presents unique challenges for caregivers. Caregivers play a vital role in providing emotional and practical support to their loved ones with leukemia. In this essay, we will discuss the resources available to caregivers of patients with leukemia.

The first step for caregivers is to educate themselves about the disease. This can include learning about the different types of leukemia, treatment options, and possible side effects. Caregivers can also learn about the patient's individual needs, including any dietary restrictions or mobility issues. Knowledge is power, and having a better understanding of leukemia can help caregivers feel more confident in their role.

Support groups are a valuable resource for caregivers. These groups provide a safe space for caregivers to share their experiences and emotions with others who are going through similar situations. Support groups can also offer practical advice and tips for managing the challenges of caregiving. Many hospitals and cancer centers offer support groups specifically for caregivers of leukemia patients.

Counseling is another resource that caregivers can utilize. Caregiving can be emotionally taxing, and it's important for caregivers to prioritize their own mental health. A mental health professional can provide guidance on coping strategies and offer a space for caregivers to process their feelings.

Respite care is a temporary relief service that allows caregivers to take a break from their caregiving duties. Respite care can be provided in a variety of settings, including in-home care, adult day care centers, or residential facilities. This service allows caregivers to take a break from their caregiving responsibilities and focus on their own needs. Respite care can also be beneficial for patients, as it provides an opportunity for socialization and engagement in activities.

Financial assistance programs are available to help offset the cost of care. These programs can provide financial assistance for medical expenses, prescription drugs, and other necessary expenses. The Leukemia & Lymphoma Society offers a financial assistance program for eligible patients and their families. Social workers or financial counselors at hospitals and cancer centers can also provide information about financial assistance programs.

Caregivers can also benefit from practical resources such as meal delivery services or transportation assistance. Many organizations provide meal delivery services for patients and caregivers, which can help alleviate the stress of meal planning and preparation. Transportation assistance can help caregivers get to and from medical appointments or other necessary errands.

In addition to these resources, caregivers can also take advantage of online resources such as blogs, forums, and websites. These resources can provide valuable information and support for caregivers who may not have access to support groups or other in-person resources. The Leukemia & Lymphoma Society and CancerCare are two examples of organizations that offer online resources for caregivers.

caregivers of leukemia patients play an important role in providing emotional and practical support to their loved ones. There are many resources available to help caregivers manage the challenges of caregiving, including support groups, counseling, respite care, financial assistance programs, and practical resources such as meal delivery and transportation assistance. Caregivers can also take advantage of online resources to connect with others and access information and support. By utilizing these resources, caregivers can provide the best possible care to their loved ones with leukemia while also prioritizing their own health and well-being.

Financial and Legal Considerations

Leukemia is a type of cancer that affects the blood and bone marrow. It can cause a variety of physical, emotional, and financial challenges for patients and their families. In addition to coping with the diagnosis and treatment of leukemia, patients and their caregivers must also deal with financial and legal considerations related to their care.

One of the main financial considerations for leukemia patients is the cost of treatment. Leukemia treatment can be very expensive, and may involve multiple hospital stays, procedures, and medications. Even with insurance coverage, patients may still be responsible for copays, deductibles, and other out-of-pocket expenses. In some cases, patients may be unable to work during treatment, which can further exacerbate financial challenges.

To help manage the financial burden of leukemia treatment, patients and their families may consider seeking financial assistance from a variety of sources. Some organizations, such as the Leukemia and Lymphoma Society, offer financial assistance programs for patients and families. Additionally, patients may be eligible for disability benefits, such as Social Security Disability Insurance, which can provide some income during treatment. It is important to research available resources and work with a financial advisor or social worker to identify and access these resources.

Another important consideration for leukemia patients and their caregivers is legal planning. This may include creating a will, assigning power of attorney, and making healthcare directives. These documents can help ensure that patients' wishes are respected in the event of incapacitation or death. Additionally, patients may want to consider appointing a financial power of attorney to manage their financial affairs during treatment.

It is also important for patients and their caregivers to understand their rights under the law. For example, patients have the right to access their medical records and to request a second opinion on their diagnosis or treatment plan. Additionally, patients have the right to file complaints or grievances with their healthcare provider or insurance company if they feel that their rights have been violated.

Emotional support is another important aspect of coping with leukemia. Patients and caregivers may experience a range of emotions, including fear, anxiety, and depression, which can impact their ability to cope with the disease. It is important to seek emotional support from loved ones, support groups, or a mental health professional. Patients may also benefit from stress-reducing activities such as exercise, meditation, or yoga.

Caregivers play a crucial role in supporting leukemia patients. They may help manage medical appointments and medications, provide emotional support, and help with daily tasks such as meal preparation and transportation. Caregivers also need support and resources to help them manage the challenges of caregiving. Support groups and respite care programs can provide caregivers with emotional support and a break from caregiving responsibilities.

leukemia can present a variety of financial and legal challenges for patients and their caregivers. It is important to be aware of available resources and to work with a financial advisor or social worker to identify and access these resources. Patients and caregivers should also prioritize emotional support and self-care to help manage the emotional impact of leukemia. Finally, caregivers should seek out support and resources to help them manage the challenges of caregiving. By addressing these issues, patients and caregivers can better manage the challenges of leukemia and improve their quality of life.

Health Insurance and Medical Expenses

Leukemia is a type of cancer that affects the blood and bone marrow, which are the spongy tissues inside the bones that produce blood cells. It is a chronic condition that requires ongoing medical care and treatment. The cost of leukemia treatment can be high, which makes it important for patients to have health insurance coverage and to understand their options for managing medical expenses.

Health insurance is a type of insurance that helps to cover the cost of medical care. There are several types of health insurance plans, including private insurance, employer-sponsored insurance, and government-sponsored insurance programs like Medicare and Medicaid. Each type of insurance plan has different coverage options and costs associated with it.

Patients with leukemia should work closely with their healthcare providers to understand the treatment options available to them and the associated costs. Treatment for leukemia typically involves a combination of chemotherapy, radiation therapy, and other medications. In addition to the cost of these treatments, patients may also need to pay for hospital stays, lab tests, imaging studies, and other medical services.

One option for managing the cost of leukemia treatment is to have health insurance coverage. Patients can purchase private health insurance plans or obtain coverage through their employer. Patients who are eligible for government-sponsored insurance programs like Medicare or Medicaid may also be able to get coverage for their medical expenses.

Health insurance plans may have different levels of coverage for leukemia treatment. Some plans may cover all or a portion of the cost of chemotherapy, radiation therapy, and other medical treatments. Other plans may have higher deductibles or copayments, which means that patients will have to pay a larger portion of the cost of their medical care out of pocket.

Patients should review their health insurance plan carefully to understand what is covered and what is not covered. They should also understand the costs associated with their plan, including deductibles, copayments, and out-of-pocket maximums. Patients who have questions about their health insurance coverage should contact their insurance provider or speak with a healthcare professional.

In addition to health insurance, there are other options for managing the cost of leukemia treatment. Patients may be eligible for financial assistance programs offered by pharmaceutical companies, nonprofit organizations, and government agencies. These programs may provide financial assistance for the cost of medication, copayments, and other medical expenses.

Patients can also speak with their healthcare providers about options for managing medical expenses. For example, some hospitals and medical centers offer payment plans that allow patients to spread out the cost of their medical care over time. Patients can also ask about options for generic medications, which are often less expensive than brand-name medications.

It is important for patients to understand their options for managing medical expenses and to work with their healthcare providers to develop a plan that works for them. Patients who are struggling to pay for their medical care should not hesitate to reach out for help. There are many resources available to assist patients with the financial and legal aspects of managing their healthcare.

health insurance and medical expenses are important considerations for patients with leukemia. Patients should review their health insurance coverage carefully and understand the costs associated with their plan. They should also explore other options for managing medical expenses, including financial assistance programs, payment plans, and generic medications. By working with their healthcare providers and taking advantage of available resources, patients can manage the financial aspects of their medical care and focus on their treatment and recovery.

Employment and Disability Rights

Leukemia is a serious and life-threatening disease that affects many individuals worldwide. It can have a significant impact on not only the patient but also their loved ones, including their ability to work and earn a living. For this reason, it's essential to understand the employment and disability rights that are available to individuals with leukemia.

Employment and disability rights refer to the legal protections that are in place to ensure that individuals with disabilities are not discriminated against in the workplace. These rights are enforced by various federal and state laws, including the Americans with Disabilities Act (ADA) and the Rehabilitation Act of 1973.

The ADA prohibits employers from discriminating against individuals with disabilities, including leukemia, in all aspects of employment, including hiring, promotions, and terminations. It also requires employers to provide reasonable accommodations to individuals with disabilities, such as modified work schedules or equipment, to enable them to perform their job duties.

The Rehabilitation Act of 1973 requires federal agencies and employers who receive federal funding to provide equal employment opportunities to individuals with disabilities, including leukemia. This law also requires these employers to provide reasonable accommodations to employees with disabilities.

In addition to these laws, individuals with leukemia may be entitled to certain benefits under the Social Security Disability Insurance (SSDI) program. SSDI is a federal program that provides financial assistance to individuals who are unable to work due to a disability.

To be eligible for SSDI, individuals must meet specific requirements, including having a condition that prevents them from working and having worked long enough to qualify for benefits. Individuals with leukemia may be eligible for SSDI if their condition is severe enough to prevent them from working for at least a year.

Individuals with leukemia may also be eligible for benefits under the Supplemental Security Income (SSI) program, which provides financial assistance to individuals with low income and limited resources. Eligibility for SSI is based on income and resource limits and disability status.

In addition to these federal programs, individuals with leukemia may be eligible for state-specific benefits, such as disability insurance or workers' compensation. It's essential to check with your state's department of labor or disability services to determine what benefits are available.

Employers may also offer disability insurance or other benefits to employees with disabilities, including leukemia. These benefits may include short-term or long-term disability insurance, paid time off, or flexible work arrangements.

It's important for individuals with leukemia and their loved ones to understand their employment and disability rights and the benefits available to them. They should also consider seeking the assistance of an attorney or disability advocate to help navigate the complex laws and regulations surrounding these issues.

individuals with leukemia face many challenges, including employment and financial difficulties. However, there are legal protections and benefits available to help alleviate some of these challenges. It's essential for individuals with leukemia and their loved ones to educate themselves about their rights and the resources available to them to ensure that they receive the support and assistance they need.

Advance Directives and Estate Planning

Advance directives and estate planning are important considerations for anyone, but they take on even greater significance for individuals with leukemia. Leukemia is a type of cancer that affects the blood and bone marrow, and it can have a significant impact on a person's health and quality of life. It is important for individuals with leukemia to plan ahead for their medical care and financial affairs, both to ensure that their wishes are respected and to relieve the burden on their loved ones.

One of the most important aspects of advance directives is the designation of a healthcare proxy or durable power of attorney for healthcare. This is a person designated to make medical decisions on behalf of the patient if they become incapacitated or are otherwise unable to make decisions for themselves. The healthcare proxy should be someone the patient trusts and who is willing and able to advocate for their wishes. It is important to discuss one's wishes for medical treatment and end-of-life care with the healthcare proxy and to ensure that they are aware of the patient's values and beliefs.

Another aspect of advance directives is the living will, which is a written document that outlines a person's preferences for medical treatment and end-of-life care. This document can provide guidance to the healthcare proxy and medical providers in situations where the patient is unable to communicate their wishes. Living wills can cover a range of topics, including resuscitation, artificial nutrition and hydration, and pain management. It is important to review and update the living will regularly to ensure that it accurately reflects the patient's current wishes.

Estate planning is also an important consideration for individuals with leukemia. This involves the preparation of legal documents that outline how a person's assets will be distributed after their death. Estate planning can include the creation of a will, which is a legal document that outlines how a person's assets will be distributed after their death. A will can also designate a guardian for any minor children and specify funeral arrangements.

In addition to a will, estate planning may also involve the creation of a trust. A trust is a legal arrangement in which a trustee holds and manages assets for the benefit of the beneficiary. Trusts can be useful in situations where the beneficiary is a minor or has special needs, as they can provide ongoing financial support while protecting the assets from creditors.

Another important consideration in estate planning is the designation of beneficiaries for life insurance policies, retirement accounts, and other financial accounts. It is important to review and update these designations regularly to ensure that they reflect the person's current wishes.

In addition to advance directives and estate planning, individuals with leukemia may also need to consider disability rights and employment issues. The Americans with Disabilities Act (ADA) provides protections for individuals with disabilities in the workplace, including accommodations for medical conditions. It is important to be aware of one's rights under the ADA and to communicate with employers about any necessary accommodations.

If the leukemia is severe enough to make it impossible for the individual to work, they may be eligible for Social Security Disability Insurance (SSDI) or Supplemental Security Income (SSI). These programs provide financial support to individuals who are unable to work due to a medical condition. It is important to work with a qualified attorney or disability advocate to navigate the application process and to ensure that all necessary documentation is provided.

Chapter Nine

Frequently Asked Questions.

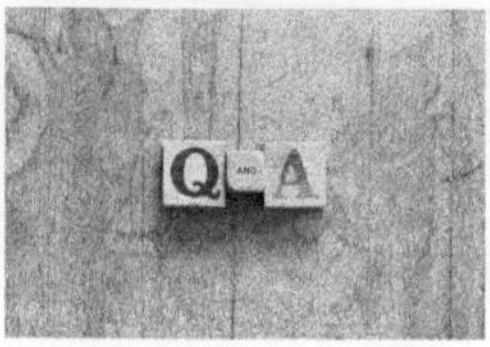

What are the first signs of having Leukemia?

The first signs of Leukemia can be easy to overlook. They may seem like nothing more than a cold or the flu. However, there are some key differences between the two that can help you telling them apart. One of the first signs of Leukemia is extreme fatigue. This fatigue doesn't go away with basic rest and can be constant. It can make everyday activities, such as going to work or school, very difficult. Another early sign of Leukemia is fever. This is generally accompanies by sweats, especially at night. The fever may come and go, but it can be a telltale sign that something more serious is going on. Leukemia can also cause weight loss and loss of appetite. This is because the cancerous cells are taking up space and nutrients that the healthy cells need. As a result, people with Leukemia may find that they're losing weight even though they're not trying to. Other early signs of Leukemia include swollen lymph nodes, easy bruising or bleeding, and feeling full even after eating a small amount. If you experience any of these signs, it's important to see a doctor so that they can rule out other potential causes and give you a proper diagnosis.

What is the survival rate of leukaemia?

According to the National Cancer Registry, the five-year survival rate for Leukemia is 63.8 percent. However, this number does not include patients who have not yet completed their treatment or who have relapsed. The five-year survival rate for those who are cured of their Leukemia is 91.3 percent. The survival rate varies depending on the type of Leukemia, with chronic lymphocytic Leukemia having the highest survival rate at 89.7 percent and acute myeloid Leukemia having the lowest at 26.8 percent. The survival rate also varies by age, with children under the age of 15 having a five-year survival rate of 83.4 percent and adults over the age of 65 having a survival rate of only 42.3 percent. Treatment for Leukemia has also improved over the years, with the five-year survival rate doubling since 1960. Leukemia is a cancer of the blood cells. The four main types of blood cells are red blood cells, which carry oxygen to the body's tissues; white blood cells, which fight infection; platelets, which help the blood to clot; and plasma, the liquid part of the blood. In Leukemia, the body produces abnormal white blood cells that do not function properly. These abnormal cells crowd out the healthy blood cells, making it difficult for the body to fight infection and affect other important functions. Leukemia can be either acute or chronic. Acute Leukemia is a fast-growing cancer that rapidly invades the blood. Chronic Leukemia is a slower-growing cancer that generally does not require immediate treatment. There are many factors that affect an individual's survival rate, including the type of Leukemia, the age of the patient, and the overall health of the patient. Treatment options have also improved over the years, with newer treatments having higher success rates.

What causes leukaemia?

There are a few different things that can cause leukaemia, but researchers are still trying to pinpoint the exact cause. Some cancers form when the body produces too many white blood cells, which crowd out the healthy blood cells. This may be the result of a genetic mutation that is passed down in families. Other times, it can be caused by something that damages the DNA in blood-forming cells, like certain chemicals or radiation. Leukaemia can also develop from other blood disorders. For example, someone with myelodysplastic syndrome (MDS) has abnormal blood cells that don't function properly. MDS can evolve into leukaemia over time. Doctors have also found that people with certain viruses, like the Epstein-Barr virus, are more likely to develop leukaemia. However, it's important to remember that most people who have these viruses don't get leukaemia. While the exact cause of leukaemia is still unknown, researchers are continuing to work to find the answer. In the meantime, there are treatments available that can help people manage the disease.

What happens when a person has Leukemia?

When a person has Leukemia, their body produces abnormal white blood cells. These abnormal cells build up in the bone marrow and blood, crowding out the healthy blood cells. This can cause a decrease in red blood cells, which can lead to fatigue and an increased risk of infection. The abnormal white blood cells can also affect the production of platelets, which are necessary for proper blood clotting. Leukemia can cause bleeding and bruising, as well as problems with the function of the immune system. In some cases, the Leukemia cells can spread to other parts of the body, such as the liver, spleen, or brain. This can cause additional symptoms, such as enlarged lymph nodes, pain in the abdomen, or headaches. Leukemia is a serious illness that can be fatal if it is not treated. There are different types of Leukemia, which are classified according to how fast the disease is progressing and which cells are affected. Treatment for Leukemia typically involves chemotherapy, which uses drugs to kill the cancer cells. In some cases, a bone marrow transplant may be necessary.

How long can you have leukaemia without knowing?

You might have leukaemia for years without knowing it. The first step in finding out if you have leukaemia is to have a blood test. From there, you might have more tests, like a bone marrow biopsy, to confirm the diagnosis. Leukaemia is cancer of the blood cells. Most blood cells form in the bone marrow, the spongy tissue inside some bones. In leukaemia, cancer cells crowd out healthy blood cells in the bone marrow. As the cancer cells grow, they might crowd out so many healthy cells that the blood cannot do its job. There are different types of leukaemia, and each type has different symptoms. Some people with leukaemia might not have any symptoms at all. But for others, leukaemia can cause fatigue, bleeding, and infections. If you have any of these symptoms, it doesn't necessarily mean you have leukaemia. But it's important to see a doctor so they can rule out other causes. If you do have leukaemia, treatment will depend on the type of leukaemia and how advanced it is. Treatment can include chemotherapy, radiation therapy, and/or a stem cell transplant. In some cases, leukaemia can be cured. But even if it can't be cured, treatment can help control the cancer and extend your life.

What are the red flags for Leukemia?

There are a few key things that can be red flags for Leukemia. One is persistent fatigue and weakness, even if you're getting enough rest. Another is easy bruising or bleeding, even from minor injuries. You might also have fever, night sweats, or weight loss. If you have any of these symptoms, it's important to see a doctor right away. They can perform tests to see if you have Leukemia, and if so, what kind of Leukemia it is. There are many different types of Leukemia, and each is treated differently. The sooner you can get a diagnosis, the sooner you can start treatment and have the best chance of a good outcome.

How long can a leukaemia patient live?

How long can a person with leukaemia live? This is often a question patients and their loved ones want to know. While understanding the average life expectancy of leukaemia patients can be helpful, it's important to remember that every individual's case is different. Some patients may only live for a few months, while others may survive for many years. According to the American Cancer Society, the 5-year survival rate for all leukaemia patients is approximately 64%. This means that 64% of people with leukaemia will live for at least 5 years after being diagnosed. However, the 10-year survival rate is only about 49%. Survival rates are generally lower for patients over the age of 60. While the 5- and 10-year survival rates provide some general information about how long leukaemia patients can live, it's important to keep in mind that these numbers don't necessarily reflect what will happen in any individual case. Some people with leukaemia will live much longer than 5 or 10 years, while others will not. There are many factors that can affect a person's life expectancy, such as the type of leukaemia they have, their age, their overall health, and how well their cancer responds to treatment. In general, patients with acute leukaemia have a better prognosis than those with chronic leukaemia. Younger patients also tend to have a better prognosis than older patients. If you or a loved one has been diagnosed with leukaemia, it's important to talk to your doctor about your specific case. They will be able to give you more information about what to expect and how long you may live.

Despite leukaemia being a cancer of the blood cells, it is still treatable and many people go on to live normal, healthy lives. There are many different types of leukaemia, which can be divided into two main groups: acute and chronic. Acute leukaemia is a rapidly progressing form of the disease that can be fatal if not treated quickly, while chronic leukaemia progresses more slowly and is less likely to be life-threatening. With advances in medical treatment, the survival rates for both types of leukaemia have increased significantly in recent years.

Is Leukemia able to be cured?

Leukemia is a cancer of the blood cells. The four main types of Leukemia are acute lymphoblastic Leukemia, chronic lymphocytic Leukemia, acute myeloid Leukemia, and chronic myeloid Leukemia. Although there are different types of Leukemia, they all have one thing in common: the uncontrolled growth of abnormal blood cells. Leukemia is treated with chemotherapy, radiation, and/or stem cell transplant. The type of treatment depends on the type of Leukemia, the age of the patient, and the health of the patient. Acute lymphoblastic Leukemia is the most common type of Leukemia in children. It is also the most treatable. The cure rate for children with acute lymphoblastic Leukemia is about 90%. Chronic lymphocytic Leukemia is the most common type of Leukemia in adults. It is a slow-growing cancer, and treatments can often keep it in check for years. There is no cure for chronic lymphocytic Leukemia, but treatments can often prolong a person's life. Acute myeloid Leukemia is a fast-growing cancer that can be difficult to treat. The cure rate for acute myeloid Leukemia is about 40%. Chronic myeloid Leukemia is a slower-growing cancer than acute myeloid Leukemia, but it is still a serious disease. There is no cure for chronic myeloid Leukemia, but treatments can often prolong a person's life. Leukemia is a serious disease, but it is treatable. The type of treatment depends on the type of Leukemia, the age of the patient, and the health of the patient. There is no one-size-fits-all treatment for Leukemia, but with the right treatment, many people with Leukemia can live long and healthy lives.

Can you suddenly get Leukemia?

Leukaemia is a type of cancer that affects the blood and bone marrow. The word 'leukaemia' actually comes from the Greek words for 'white' (leukos) and 'blood' (haima). This is because in people with leukaemia, the cancer cells prevent the bone marrow from making normal, healthy blood cells. Leukaemia can develop suddenly, but it is more often a gradual process. In most cases, leukaemia is not hereditary, which means it is not passed down from generation to generation in families. However, there are a small number of cases where leukaemia is linked to an inherited gene mutation. There are four main types of leukaemia: • Acute lymphoblastic leukaemia (ALL) • Acute myeloid leukaemia (AML) • Chronic lymphocytic leukaemia (CLL) • Chronic myeloid leukaemia (CML) The type of leukaemia someone has will determine their symptoms and the course of their disease. Leukaemia is most commonly diagnosed in adults over the age of 55, but it can affect people of all ages. In fact, leukaemia is the most common cancer in children under the age of 15. There are many different symptoms of leukaemia, and they can vary depending on the type of leukaemia someone has. Some common symptoms include: • Feeling tired all the time • Shortness of breath • Easy bruising or bleeding • Fever • Weight loss • Pain in the bones or joints • swellings in the neck, armpits, or groin •Repeated infections If you experience any of these symptoms, it is important to see your doctor as soon as possible. Early diagnosis and treatment of leukaemia is crucial for the best possible outcome.

Where does Leukemia usually begin?

Leukemia is a cancer of the blood cells. It is the most common type of cancer in children, but can also affect adults. Most Leukemias start in the bone marrow, the soft tissue inside bones where blood cells are made. Leukemia happens when something goes wrong in the process of making blood cells. In Leukemia, the bone marrow produces abnormal white blood cells. These cells crowd out the healthy blood cells, making it difficult for the body to fight infection. The abnormal cells can also spread to other parts of the body, such as the lymph nodes, liver, and brain. There are four main types of Leukemia, based on how quickly the disease develops and the type of blood cell that is affected. The four types are: -Acute lymphoblastic Leukemia (ALL): This is the most common type of Leukemia in children. It can also occur in adults, but is less common. ALL develops quickly and affects the white blood cells called lymphocytes. -Acute myeloid Leukemia (AML): AML is the most common type of Leukemia in adults. It can also occur in children, but is less common. AML develops quickly and affects the white blood cells called myelocytes. -Chronic lymphocytic Leukemia (CLL): CLL is the most common type of Leukemia in adults. It develops slowly and affects the white blood cells called lymphocytes. -Chronic myeloid Leukemia (CML): CML is less common than the other types of Leukemia. It develops slowly and affects the white blood cells called myelocytes. Leukemia is treated with chemotherapy, radiation, and/or bone marrow transplant. The type of treatment depends on the type of Leukemia and how advanced it is.

Is Leukemia curable if caught early?

Leukemia is a cancer of the blood cells. The four main types of Leukemia are acute lymphoblastic Leukemia (ALL), chronic lymphocytic Leukemia (CLL), acute myeloid Leukemia (AML), and chronic myeloid Leukemia (CML). Leukemia is treated with chemotherapy, radiation therapy, and sometimes stem cell transplant. The chances of a cure depend on the type of Leukemia, the stage of the cancer, the patient's age and general health, and other factors. In general, the outlook is better for children and young adults than for older adults. Acute lymphoblastic Leukemia (ALL) is the most common type of Leukemia in children. It is also called acute lymphocytic Leukemia. With treatment, about 80% of children with ALL can be cured. Chronic lymphocytic Leukemia (CLL) is the most common type of Leukemia in adults. In the past, CLL was considered a cancer that could not be cured. But with newer treatments, People with CLL now can live for many years with the disease and die from other causes. Acute myeloid Leukemia (AML) is a cancer that starts in the bone marrow. In the past, only about one-third of people with AML could be cured. With newer treatments, the cure rate has improved to 40% to 50%. Chronic myeloid Leukemia (CML) is cancer that starts in the bone marrow. In the past, CML was considered a cancer that could not be cured. But with newer treatments, People with CML now can live for many years with the disease and die from other causes.

What age is Leukemia most common?

Leukemia is most common in adults over the age of 55, although it can occur at any age. The average age of diagnosis is 64. Leukemia is more common in men than in women, and the incidence increases with age. There are four main types of Leukemia, which are classified according to the type of blood cell that is affected: lymphoblastic, myeloid, monocytic and erythroid. Lymphoblastic Leukemia is the most common type of Leukemia in children, accounting for around three quarters of all cases. It usually affects young children, with the average age of diagnosis being 6. Myeloid Leukemia is the most common type of Leukemia in adults, accounting for around two thirds of all cases. It usually affects adults over the age of 55, with the average age of diagnosis being 64. Monocytic Leukemia is a rare type of Leukemia that accounts for less than 5% of all cases. It usually affects adults over the age of 55, with the average age of diagnosis being 67. Erythroid Leukemia is the rarest type of Leukemia, accounting for less than 1% of all cases. It usually affects adults over the age of 55, with the average age of diagnosis being 70. Leukemia is a cancer of the blood cells. The four main types of blood cells are red blood cells, white blood cells, platelets and lymphocytes. Red blood cells carry oxygen around the body. White blood cells fight infection. Platelets help to stop bleeding. Lymphocytes are a type of white blood cell that helps to fight infection. There are three main types of lymphocytes: B-cells, T-cells and natural killer cells. B-cells make antibodies, which are proteins that fight infection. T-cells kill viruses and cancer cells. Natural killer cells kill cancer cells. Leukemia occurs when the DNA of a blood cell is damaged. This damage can be caused by exposure to ionizing radiation, chemicals or viruses. The damaged blood cell then starts to grow and divide uncontrollably. The resulting abnormal cells are less effective at fighting infection and are also more likely to break down and die. This can lead to a build-up of abnormal cells in the blood, known as Leukemia. There are four main types of Leukemia, which are classified according to the type of blood cell that is affected: lymphoblastic, myeloid, monocytic and erythroid. Lymphoblastic Leukemia is the most common type of Leukemia in children, accounting for around three quarters of all cases. It usually affects young children, with the average age of diagnosis being 6. Myeloid Leukemia is the most common type of Leukemia in adults, accounting for around two thirds of all cases. It usually affects adults over the age of 55, with the average age of diagnosis being 64. Monocytic Leukemia is a rare type of Leukemia that accounts for less than 5% of all cases

Would Leukemia show up in blood test?

Leukemia is a cancer of the blood cells. The most common type of Leukemia in adults is called chronic lymphocytic Leukemia (CLL). In

CLL, the Leukemia cells build up in the bone marrow and crowd out the healthy blood cells. The Leukemia cells may also build up in the lymph nodes and other parts of the body. The symptoms of Leukemia may not appear until the Leukemia has reached an advanced stage. When symptoms do appear, they may include: - fatigue - easy bruising or bleeding - shortness of breath - weight loss - bone pain or tenderness If you have any of these symptoms, it is important to see your doctor so that he or she can order the appropriate tests. One of the tests that may be ordered is a blood test. A blood test can help to diagnose Leukemia. The test can show if there are too many white blood cells or too few red blood cells or platelets in the blood. The blood test can also help to determine which type of Leukemia you have. If you are diagnosed with Leukemia, your doctor will discuss treatment options with you. Treatment for Leukemia may include: - chemotherapy - radiation therapy - targeted therapy - stem cell transplant Your doctor will recommend the best treatment for you based on the type of Leukemia you have, your age, your overall health, and your preferences.

Who is most likely to get Leukemia?

Leukemia is a type of cancer that begins in the blood-forming cells of the bone marrow. The bone marrow is the spongy tissue inside some of the bones of the body, where blood cells are made. Leukemia may affect people of any age, but is most common in children and older adults. In the United States, Leukemia is the cancer that most often affects children younger than 15 years old. It is also the cancer that most often affects adults older than 55 years old. Certain factors may increase a person's risk of developing Leukemia. These include: * Previous cancer treatment with certain drugs or radiation * A family history of Leukemia * Exposure to certain chemicals, such as benzene * Having certain blood disorders, such as polycythemia vera or myelodysplastic syndromes * A weakened immune system There is no sure way to prevent Leukemia. But you may be able to lower your risk by avoiding known risk factors, such as exposure to certain chemicals. You may also be able to lower your risk by taking steps to boost your immune system.

Leukaemia is a serious medical condition that can be life-threatening. Early diagnosis and treatment is essential for the best possible outcome.

What can be confused for Leukemia?

There are many forms of Leukemia, and the symptoms can vary depending on the type. It is important to see a doctor if you think you may have Leukemia, as some of the symptoms can be confused for other conditions. One type of Leukemia is acute lymphoblastic Leukemia (ALL). The symptoms of ALL can include fatigue, fever, weight loss, easy bruising or bleeding, and bone or joint pain. These symptoms can be caused by other conditions, so it is important to see a doctor if you are experiencing any of them. Chronic lymphocytic Leukemia (CLL) is another type of Leukemia. The symptoms of CLL can be similar to those of ALL, but they may also include itching, enlarged lymph nodes, and night sweats. Again, these symptoms can be caused by other conditions, so it is important to see a doctor if you are experiencing any of them. Leukemia can also be confused with other blood disorders, such as anemia. Anemia can cause fatigue, pale skin, and shortness of breath. However, anemia is usually not accompanied by fever, easy bruising or bleeding, or bone or joint pain. If you are experiencing any of these symptoms, it is important to see a doctor to rule out Leukemia. There are many other conditions that can cause symptoms that are similar to those of Leukemia. This is why it is so important to see a doctor if you are experiencing any of the symptoms of Leukemia. Only a doctor can properly diagnose Leukemia.

How fatal is Leukemia?

Leukemia is a cancer of the blood cells. The four main types of Leukemia are acute lymphoblastic Leukemia (ALL), acute myeloid Leukemia (AML), chronic lymphocytic Leukemia (CLL) and chronic myeloid Leukemia (CML). Leukemia can be either fatal or non-fatal. The majority of Leukemia cases are non-fatal. In fact, the five-year survival rate for Leukemia is 65%. However, this does not mean that all patients will survive for five years after diagnosis. The five-year survival rate simply means that out of 100 patients diagnosed with Leukemia, 65 will still be alive five years later. So how fatal is Leukemia? It depends on the type of Leukemia. For ALL, the five-year survival rate is 87%. For AML, the five-year survival rate is 40%. For CLL, the five-year survival rate is 83%. For CML, the five-year survival rate is 60%. As you can see, the survival rate varies depending on the type of Leukemia. Leukemia is a serious disease and it can be fatal. However, the survival rate has increased over the years thanks to advances in treatment and early detection. If you have been diagnosed with Leukemia, it is important to talk to your doctor about your prognosis and treatment options.

Can you live a full life after Leukemia?

Leukemia is a cancer of the blood cells. The four main types of Leukemia are lymphocytic, myelogenous, monocytic, and erythroblastic. In general, treatment for Leukemia involves chemotherapy, radiation therapy, and stem cell transplant. The type of Leukemia, as well as the stage of the disease, determines the best course of treatment. Although Leukemia is a serious illness, many people with Leukemia can expect to lead long, full lives. With advances in treatment, the survival rate for Leukemia has increased dramatically in recent years. In fact, the 5-year survival rate for Leukemia has increased from 24 percent in 1960 to 61 percent in 2010. Of course, living with Leukemia does come with challenges. Many people experience side effects from treatment, such as fatigue, nausea, and hair loss. It can be difficult to cope with the emotional toll of the disease. However, there are many resources available to help people manage their Leukemia and its effects. If you or someone you love has been diagnosed with Leukemia, it is important to remember that there is hope. With proper treatment, many people with Leukemia can lead long, full lives.

Is Leukemia always terminal?

Leukemia is a cancer of the blood cells. The four main types of Leukemia are acute lymphoblastic Leukemia, acute myeloid Leukemia, chronic lymphocytic Leukemia, and chronic myeloid Leukemia. Leukemia is often described as a cancer of the blood, but it actually starts in the bone marrow. The bone marrow is the spongy tissue inside the bones where blood cells are made. In Leukemia, something goes wrong with the bone marrow so that it starts making abnormal blood cells. Most types of Leukemia can be treated, but some are harder to treat than others. The outlook depends on the type of Leukemia and how early it is found. Acute Leukemia is the most common type of Leukemia in children, but it can also occur in adults. Acute Leukemia is a fast-growing type of Leukemia that can be life-threatening if not treated right away. Chronic Leukemia grows more slowly and is common in older adults. People with chronic Leukemia may not have any symptoms for months or even years. In general, Leukemia that starts in children (acute lymphoblastic Leukemia and acute myeloid Leukemia) is easier to treat than Leukemia that starts in adults (chronic lymphocytic Leukemia and chronic myeloid Leukemia). This is because children's bodies can usually tolerate more aggressive treatment than adults. Most people with Leukemia can be cured with treatment. The goal of treatment is to keep the Leukemia from spreading and to allow the bone marrow to make normal blood cells. The type of treatment depends on the type of Leukemia. Treatment for Leukemia can bemlasti divided into two types: local therapy and systemic therapy. Local therapy treats the Leukemia cells in one specific area of the body. Systemic therapy treats the whole body. Local therapy for Leukemia can be either radiation therapy or surgery. Radiation therapy uses high-energy beams to kill cancer cells. Surgery removes the Leukemia cells from the body. Systemic therapy for Leukemia can be either chemotherapy or targeted therapy. Chemotherapy uses drugs to kill cancer cells. Targeted therapy uses drugs that target specific genes or proteins in cancer cells. Is Leukemia always terminal? No, Leukemia is not always terminal. With treatment, most people with Leukemia can be cured. The goal of treatment is to keep the Leukemia from spreading and to allow the bone marrow to make normal blood cells. The type of treatment depends on the type of Leukemia.

How successful is chemotherapy for Leukemia?

Around 70% of people with leukaemia will achieve remission with chemotherapy. remission is when the cancerous cells in your body decrease to the point where they can no longer be detected. However, this does not necessarily mean that the cancer is cured and it is still possible for the cancer to come back. If the cancer does come back, it is often possible to treat it again with chemotherapy. However, each time the cancer comes back, it is more difficult to treat. There are many different types of leukaemia, and each responds differently to chemotherapy. The most common type of leukaemia, acute lymphoblastic leukaemia (ALL), is usually very responsive to chemotherapy. Around 85% of people with ALL will achieve remission with chemotherapy. Chronic lymphocytic leukaemia (CLL) is the second most common type of leukaemia. It often responds well to chemotherapy, but the cancer can become resistant over time. Around 65% of people with CLL will achieve remission with chemotherapy. Acute myeloid leukaemia (AML) is the third most common type of leukaemia. It is usually more difficult to treat than ALL or CLL. Around 50% of people with AML will achieve remission with chemotherapy. There are many side effects of chemotherapy that can range from mild to severe. The most common side effects are fatigue, nausea and vomiting, hair loss, and increased risk of infection. These side effects usually go away once treatment is finished. Some people may experience more severe side effects from chemotherapy, such as heart or kidney damage, or problems with their nervous system. These side effects are more likely to occur with certain types of chemotherapy drugs. It is important to talk to your doctor about the risks and side effects of chemotherapy before starting treatment.

What is lemons for Leukemia?

Lemons are a type of citrus fruit that are thought to be beneficial for people with Leukemia. While there is no cure for Leukemia, some evidence suggests that lemons may help to improve the symptoms and prognosis of the disease. Lemons are a good source of vitamin C, which is a nutrient that is essential for immune system function. Additionally, lemons contain flavonoids, which are plant-based compounds that have been shown to have anti-cancer properties. There are several ways that lemons may help to treat or improve the symptoms of Leukemia. First, the vitamin C in lemons may help to boost the immune system, making it better able to fight off infection. Additionally, the flavonoids in lemons may help to kill cancer cells or stop them from growing. Finally, the acidic nature of lemons may help to improve the absorption of chemotherapy drugs, making them more effective at treating Leukemia. Although lemons may offer some benefits for people with Leukemia, it is important to remember that they are not a cure. Lemons should be used in addition to, not instead of, traditional medical treatment. If you are interested in using lemons to treat your Leukemia, be sure to speak with your doctor first to ensure that it is safe for you to do so.

Can Leukemia be inherited?

Leukemia is a cancer of the blood cells. The three main types of blood cells are red blood cells, white blood cells, and platelets. The most common type of Leukemia is acute lymphocytic Leukemia (ALL), which starts in the white blood cells. In ALL, the body makes too many abnormal lymphocytes (a type of white blood cell). The abnormal cells crowd out the normal blood cells, making it hard for the body to fight infection. Leukemia can be either inherited or acquired. Inherited Leukemia is caused by mutations (changes) in the genes that control blood cell production. These changes are passed down from parent to child. Acquired Leukemia is not inherited. It is caused by changes in the blood cells that occur during a person's lifetime. These changes happen randomly and are not passed down from parent to child. Inherited Leukemia is rare. It accounts for only a small number of all cases of Leukemia. The most common type of inherited Leukemia is familial platelet disorder with associated myeloid malignancy (FPD/AML). FPD/AML is a disorder that affects both white blood cells and platelets. People with FPD/AML have a higher than normal risk of developing Leukemia. Acquired Leukemia is much more common than inherited Leukemia. The most common type of acquired Leukemia is acute myeloid Leukemia (AML). AML starts in the myeloid cells, which are a type of white blood cell. In AML, the body makes too many abnormal myeloid cells. The abnormal cells crowd out the normal blood cells, making it hard for the body to fight infection. There are many other types of Leukemia, both inherited and acquired. Treatment for Leukemia depends on the type of Leukemia, the stage of the disease, and the person's age and health.

Leukaemia is a type of cancer that starts in the blood-forming cells of the bone marrow. The four main types of leukaemia are acute lymphoblastic leukaemia (ALL), chronic lymphoblastic leukaemia (CLL), acute myeloid leukaemia (AML) and chronic myeloid leukaemia (CML). Leukaemia can be treated with chemotherapy, radiation therapy, targeted therapy or stem cell transplant. The prognosis for leukaemia depends on the type of leukaemia, the stage of the disease, the age of the patient and other factors.

How serious is lymphocytic Leukemia?

Lymphocytic Leukemia is a cancer that starts in the white blood cells, which are an important part of the body's immune system. The cancerous cells might crowd out the normal white blood cells, making it harder for the body to fight infection. Lymphocytic Leukemia is considered to be a serious cancer, but it is also a very treatable cancer. In most cases, lymphocytic Leukemia can be cured with chemotherapy. In some cases, a bone marrow transplant might be necessary.

Is lymphocytic Leukemia curable?

Is lymphocytic Leukemia curable? Lymphocytic Leukemia is a type of blood cancer that begins in the lymphocytes, which are a type of white blood cell. The Leukemia cells grow in the bone marrow and crowd out the healthy blood cells. Lymphocytic Leukemia is the most common type of Leukemia in adults. The cause of lymphocytic Leukemia is unknown. However, there are certain risk factors that may increase your chance of developing the disease. These include being over the age of 55, having a family history of Leukemia, being exposed to certain chemicals, and having certain genetic disorders. Lymphocytic Leukemia is usually treated with chemotherapy. However, some people may also need a stem cell transplant. The treatment plan will be determined by the stage of the disease, the patient's age, and overall health. In most cases, lymphocytic Leukemia is a chronic disease. This means that it can be managed, but not cured. However, some people may go into remission, which means that there are no active Leukemia cells in the body. Remission can be temporary or permanent. Although lymphocytic Leukemia is a serious disease, there are treatments available that can help people live long and healthy lives.

What is the survival rate of lymphocytic Leukemia?

Lymphocytic Leukemia is a type of cancer that starts in the cells that become lymphocytes, which are a type of white blood cell. The survival rate for this type of Leukemia varies depending on the stage of the disease, the age of the patient, and other factors. In general, the five-year survival rate for lymphocytic Leukemia is about 60%. This means that 60% of people who are diagnosed with this type of Leukemia are still alive five years after their diagnosis. However, the survival rate is different for each stage of the disease. The survival rate for people with early-stage lymphocytic Leukemia is higher than the survival rate for people with late-stage lymphocytic Leukemia. The five-year survival rate for early-stage disease is about 80%, while the five-year survival rate for late-stage disease is about 40%. The stage of the disease is determined by how far the cancer has spread in the body. Early-stage disease is cancer that is only in the blood and bone marrow, while late-stage disease is cancer that has spread to other parts of the body, such as the liver or spleen. Age is another factor that affects the survival rate for lymphocytic Leukemia. The five-year survival rate for children under the age of 15 is about 80%. For adults over the age of 65, the five-year survival rate is about 50%. The survival rate is also higher for people who are treated with chemotherapy and radiation therapy, compared to people who are not treated with these therapies. There are many different factors that can affect the survival rate for lymphocytic Leukemia. The stage of the disease, the age of the patient, and the treatment that the patient receives are all important factors.

What causes lymphocytic Leukemia?

Lymphocytic Leukemia is a type of cancer that starts in the cells that make up the lymph system. The lymph system is part of the immune system, which helps the body fight off infections. Lymphocytes are a type of white blood cell that is found in the lymph system. There are two main types of lymphocytic Leukemia: acute lymphocytic Leukemia (ALL) and chronic lymphocytic Leukemia (CLL). Both types of Leukemia can be serious, but treatment for ALL is usually more successful. The cause of lymphocytic Leukemia is not known. However, there are some risk factors that may make a person more likely to develop the disease. These include: - Age: The risk of developing CLL increases with age. Most cases are diagnosed in people over the age of 55. - Gender: Men are more likely than women to develop CLL. - Family history: People with a family history of CLL are at an increased risk of developing the disease. - Smoking: Smoking is a risk factor for CLL. - Exposure to certain chemicals: Exposure to certain chemicals, such as benzene, may increase the risk of developing CLL. There is no sure way to prevent lymphocytic Leukemia. However, avoiding exposure to known risk factors may help reduce the risk.

Is lymphocytic Leukemia terminal?

Lymphocytic Leukemia is a type of cancer that affects the lymphocytes, which are a type of white blood cell. The cancerous cells multiply in an uncontrolled way, crowding out the normal cells. This can make it difficult for the body to fight infection and can lead to serious problems such as anaemia and bleeding. Lymphocytic Leukemia can be either acute or chronic. Acute lymphocytic Leukemia is a more aggressive form of the disease and is often fatal, whereas chronic lymphocytic Leukemia is a slower-progressing form of the disease and can be treated with medication.

Can you have Leukemia for years without knowing?

Leukemia is a cancer of the blood cells. The four main types of Leukemia are acute lymphocytic Leukemia (ALL), acute myelogenous Leukemia (AML), chronic lymphocytic Leukemia (CLL), and chronic myelogenous Leukemia (CML). Leukemia can occur in people of any age, but it is most common in children and older adults. Leukemia is usually a disease that develops over time, with symptoms worsening gradually. In some cases, however, people may not experience any symptoms for years. This is often the case with chronic Leukemias, which tend to develop more slowly than acute Leukemias. As Leukemia progresses, it can cause a wide range of symptoms, some of which are specific to the type of Leukemia. Common symptoms of Leukemia include fatigue, fever,weight loss, enlarged lymph nodes, night sweats, and easy bruising or bleeding. Leukemia can also cause more general symptoms, such as weakness and fatigue. In most cases, Leukemia is diagnosed after a person seeks medical attention for these symptoms. However, it is possible for Leukemia to be diagnosed during a routine blood test or physical exam. If Leukemia is suspected, a doctor will order additional tests, such as a bone marrow biopsy, to confirm the diagnosis. While there is no cure for Leukemia, it is treatable. The type of treatment will depend on the type of Leukemia, as well as the person's age and overall health. In many cases, treatment can lead to remission, which is when the Leukemia cells are no longer present in the body. With treatment, most people with Leukemia can expect to live long, healthy lives.

What is the best treatment for lymphocytic Leukemia?

Lymphocytic Leukemia is a type of cancer that starts in the cells that become lymphocytes in the bone marrow. Lymphocytes are a type of white blood cell that helps fight infection. In lymphocytic Leukemia, too many lymphocytes are produced. These abnormal lymphocytes crowd out the healthy blood cells in the bone marrow. They also build up in the lymph nodes and other organs. Lymphocytic Leukemia is the most common type of Leukemia in adults. It is also called chronic lymphocytic Leukemia (CLL). There are different types of treatment for lymphocytic Leukemia. The type of treatment depends on the stage of the cancer and how fast it is growing. Treatment may also depend on your age and overall health. The main treatments are: - Chemotherapy - Targeted therapy - Radiation therapy - Stem cell transplant Chemotherapy is the use of drugs to kill cancer cells. It is a systemic therapy, which means it enters the bloodstream and can reach cancer cells throughout the body. Targeted therapy is the use of drugs that target specific molecules inside cancer cells. These molecules help cancer cells grow, divide, and spread. Radiation therapy is the use of high-energy beams, such as X-rays, to kill cancer cells. A stem cell transplant is a procedure to replace your diseased bone marrow with healthy stem cells. Stem cells are the cells in the bone marrow that make all the blood cells. The decision about which type of treatment is best for you is made by a team of specialists who consider all of these factors. Clinical trials are also an important part of treatment. Clinical trials are research studies that test new treatments. You and your doctor will work together to make the best decision about your treatment.

Though leukaemia is a serious and life-threatening illness, there are treatments available that can improve the quality and length of life for patients. With continued research, even better treatments and cure rates are possible in the future.

What kills people with CLL?

Cancer is a deadly disease that claimed the lives of many people each year. One type of cancer that is particularly deadly is CLL, or chronic lymphocytic Leukemia. CLL is a form of cancer that affects the white blood cells, and it is often difficult to treat. There are many different factors that can contribute to the death of a patient with CLL, but the most common cause of death is infection. CLL cells build up in the bone marrow and the lymph nodes, crowding out the healthy cells. This can make it difficult for the body to fight off infection. patients with CLL are also at an increased risk for developing other infections, such as sepsis. This is a life-threatening condition that occurs when an infection spreads throughout the body. Other infections that can be deadly for patients with CLL include pneumonia and influenza. Cancer treatment can be very difficult, and sometimes it is not possible to save the life of a patient with CLL. Chemotherapy is often used to treat CLL, but it can have many side effects. In some cases, stem cell transplants are used to treat CLL. This is a very aggressive treatment that can have serious side effects, but it may be the only way to save the life of a patient with CLL. No matter what treatment is used, CLL is a very serious disease with a high mortality rate. The disease is often slowly progressive, and it can take years for it to reach a point where it is deadly. However, with the right treatment and care, patients with CLL can live long and healthy lives.

What is the average age of CLL patients?

CLL is a type of leukaemia that predominantly affects older people, with the median age at diagnosis being 72 years old. The average age of CLL patients is therefore likely to be slightly higher than this. However, it is important to note that CLL can affect people of all ages, with the youngest reported case being just 12 years old. CLL is a slowly progressing disease, which means that many people live with it for many years without experiencing any symptoms. In fact, around 25% of people with CLL will never need treatment. For those who do require treatment, the average life expectancy is around 10 years. However, it is important to remember that these are just averages, and that everyone's experience of CLL will be different. Some people will have a more aggressive form of the disease and will need treatment sooner, while others will have a more slowly progressing form and may not need treatment at all. There is no one-size-fits-all when it comes to CLL, and treatment decisions should be made on an individual basis.

Is lymphocytic Leukemia an autoimmune disease?

Lymphocytic Leukemia is a type of cancer that starts in the cells that make up the immune system. The immune system is made up of different types of cells, each with a specific function. One type of cell, the lymphocyte, is important for fighting infection. Lymphocytic Leukemia occurs when there is an overgrowth of lymphocytes in the blood and bone marrow. This overgrowth Crowds out other important blood cells, making it difficult for the body to fight infection. There is some evidence that lymphocytic Leukemia may be an autoimmune disease. Autoimmune diseases occur when the body's immune system attacks healthy cells by mistake. In the case of lymphocytic Leukemia, the body may produce antibodies that attack the healthy lymphocytes. This can cause the lymphocytes to die or to become abnormal. There is still much unknown about lymphocytic Leukemia, and whether or not it is an autoimmune disease. However, the fact that the body's immune system may be attacking healthy cells is an important clue that needs to be explored further.

What is the meaning of lymphocytic?

Lymphocytic refers to a type of cancer that affects the lymphocytes, which are a type of white blood cell. The lymphocytes are important for fighting infection, so when they are not functioning properly, it can lead to serious health problems. There are two main types of lymphocytic cancer:

Hodgkin lymphoma and non-Hodgkin lymphoma. Both of these types are serious and can be life-threatening.

Where does Leukemia start in the body?

Leukemia is a cancer of the blood and bone marrow. The bone marrow is the spongy tissue inside bones where blood cells are made. Leukemia can start in any blood-forming cell, but starts most often in the cells of the bone marrow. In Leukemia, the bone marrow produces abnormal white blood cells. The Leukemia cells can crowd out the normal blood cells, making it difficult for the body to get the oxygen and nutrients it needs. The abnormal cells can also invade other tissues, including the lymph nodes, liver, and brain. Leukemia is a cancer that starts in the blood-forming cells of the bone marrow. The bone marrow is the spongy tissue inside bones where blood cells are made. In Leukemia, the bone marrow produces abnormal white blood cells. The Leukemia cells can crowd out the normal blood cells, making it difficult for the body to get the oxygen and nutrients it needs. The abnormal cells can also invade other tissues, including the lymph nodes, liver, and brain. Leukemia is a serious illness, but treatment can often control the disease. With treatment, many people with Leukemia live long and healthy lives.

What are the stages of lymphocytic Leukemia?

Lymphocytic Leukemia is a type of Leukemia, a cancer of the blood cells, that starts in the cells that become lymphocytes. There are four main types of lymphocytes: B cells, T cells, natural killer (NK) cells, and null cells. Lymphocytic Leukemia can start in any of these cell types, but most often starts in B cells. Lymphocytic Leukemia is divided into two main types: chronic lymphocytic Leukemia (CLL) and acute lymphocytic Leukemia (ALL). CLL is the most common type of lymphocytic Leukemia in adults, while ALL is the most common type in children. Lymphocytic Leukemia is a slowly progressing disease. In many cases, people with CLL live for many years without symptoms and do not need treatment. For people with ALL, treatment is usually successful in achieving remission, which is when there are no signs of cancer. However, both CLL and ALL can come back after treatment, and both can be difficult to control. The stages of lymphocytic Leukemia are not well defined. The course of the disease can vary from person to person. In general, CLL progresses slowly, while ALL can progress quickly. There are four main types of treatment for lymphocytic Leukemia: chemotherapy, immunotherapy, targeted therapy, and stem cell transplant. Chemotherapy is the most common treatment for both CLL and ALL. Immunotherapy and targeted therapy are newer treatments that are becoming more common, especially for CLL. Stem cell transplant is a more aggressive treatment that is usually only used for people with ALL who do not respond to other treatments.

What are signs that CLL is progressing?

CLL is a cancer of the blood cells that typically progresses slowly. However, there are a few signs that may indicate that the disease is progressing. One sign that CLL is progressing is an increase in the number of lymphocytes in the blood. Lymphocytes are a type of white blood cell that is made in the bone marrow. In CLL, the body produces too many lymphocytes, which crowd out other blood cells and leads to a build-up in the lymph nodes. Another sign that CLL is progressing is a decrease in the number of platelets in the blood. Platelets are cells that help to clot the blood and prevent bleeding. A decrease in platelets can cause easy bruising and bleeding. Another sign of CLL progression is fatigue. This is due to the fact that the cancerous cells crowd out the healthy blood cells, leading to a decrease in oxygen and nutrients being delivered to the body's tissues. If you are experiencing any of these signs, it is important to speak to your doctor so that they can monitor the disease and provide treatment if necessary.

In conclusion, leukaemia is a type of cancer that can affect people of all ages. It is important to be aware of the symptoms of leukaemia and to see a doctor if you have any concerns. There is no one cause of leukaemia, but it is thought to be caused by a combination of genetic and environmental factors. There is no cure for leukaemia, but treatment can help to manage the disease and extend a person's life.

Can blood test detect Leukemia?

A blood test is often the first step in diagnosing Leukemia. It can help find cancer cells in the body and show how well the body is making new blood cells. There are many different types of Leukemia, and each one affects the blood cells differently. This means that not all blood tests will be able to detect all types of Leukemia. Doctors will often use other tests, such as a bone marrow biopsy, to confirm a diagnosis of Leukemia.

Is lymphocytic Leukemia painful?

There are many different types of Leukemia, and each type can cause different symptoms. lymphocytic Leukemia is a type of Leukemia that can cause pain in the bones, joints, or abdomen. The pain is often described as a dull ache. In some cases, the pain can be severe enough to interfere with daily activities. Pain is not always a symptom of Leukemia, but it can be a sign that the disease is getting worse. If you are experiencing pain, it is important to talk to your doctor so that they can determine the cause and provide treatment.

Can I live a normal life with CLL?

Cancer can be a difficult journey, and Leukemia is one type that comes with its own challenges. Leukemia is a cancer of the blood and bone marrow, which can make treatment difficult. The good news is that many people with Leukemia can live full, normal lives. There are different types of Leukemia, and the type you have will affect your treatment and outlook. Some types of Leukemia are more common in children, while others are more common in adults. Chronic lymphocytic Leukemia (CLL) is the most common type of Leukemia in adults. CLL is a slow-growing type of Leukemia, which means that symptoms may not appear for years. When symptoms do appear, they can be mild, and may include fatigue, weight loss, and easy bruising or bleeding. Because CLL grows slowly, treatment may not be necessary right away. If you are diagnosed with CLL, your doctor will likely monitor your condition with regular blood tests and bone marrow biopsies. Treatment may be necessary if the Leukemia progresses or if you experience symptoms. There are several treatment options for CLL, including chemotherapy, targeted therapy, and radiation therapy. Your doctor will work with you to choose the best treatment for your individual situation. With treatment, many people with CLL can live long, healthy lives. CLL does not have to dictate how you live your life. You can still work, travel, and do the things you enjoy. Leukemia can be a difficult journey, but you don't have to go through it alone. There are many resources available to help you and your family cope with a diagnosis of Leukemia. You can find support groups, counseling, and educational resources to help you navigate your journey.

What happens if chronic lymphocytic Leukemia is left untreated?

Chronic lymphocytic Leukemia (CLL) is a type of cancer that affects the blood and bone marrow. It is a slowly progressing form of Leukemia, and if left untreated, it can lead to serious health complications. CLL is caused by the overproduction of abnormal lymphocytes, a type of white blood cell. These abnormal cells crowd out the healthy blood cells, resulting in a lower number of healthy blood cells. This can lead to anemia, bleeding problems, and increased susceptibility to infection. If CLL is left untreated, it can progress to a more serious form of cancer, such as acute lymphoblastic Leukemia. This is a very aggressive form of Leukemia that is difficult to treat. It can be fatal if not caught early and treated effectively. CLL can also cause the lymph nodes to swell, which can lead to pain and difficulty breathing. The spleen may also become enlarged, and this can cause abdominal pain and discomfort. left untreated, CLL can be a very serious condition. It is important to see a doctor if you think you may have CLL, so that you can be diagnosed and treated early.

Can I drink alcohol with CLL?

No definitive answer exists as to whether or not patients with CLL can safely drink alcohol. Some doctors believe that alcohol consumption may exacerbate the symptoms of CLL, while others believe that moderate drinking may actually be beneficial for patients. It is generally recommended that patients with CLL avoid drinking alcohol, as it can potentially worsen the disease. Alcohol consumption can lead to dehydration, which can worsen the fatigue and other symptoms associated with CLL. In addition, alcohol can also interfere with the medications used to treat CLL, making them less effective. However, some studies have suggested that moderate alcohol consumption may actually be beneficial for patients with CLL. One study found that moderate drinkers were less likely to develop the disease than those who abstained from alcohol entirely. Another study found that moderate drinking was associated with a lower risk of death from CLL. Ultimately, the decision of whether or not to drink alcohol while living with CLL is a personal one. Patients should speak with their doctor to get the best advice for their individual situation.

What is the most common cause of death in CLL?

The most common cause of death in CLL is the development of complications related to the disease. These can include problems with the blood, such as anemia or bleeding, as well as infections. In many cases, death occurs when the disease progresses to a more advanced stage and the patient is unable to receive treatment. While there is no cure for CLL, early diagnosis and treatment can improve the chances of survival.

What is the best vitamin for CLL?

CLL, or chronic lymphocytic Leukemia, is a type of cancer that affects the blood and bone marrow. The best vitamin for CLL is vitamin C, which is an antioxidant that helps to protect cells from damage. Vitamin C also helps to boost the immune system, which can help to fight off infection.

Leukaemia is a type of cancer that affects the blood and bone marrow. It is a serious and life-threatening disease that can be difficult to treat. However, with the right treatment and support, many people with leukaemia can go on to live long and healthy lives.

What is survival rate for AML?

The overall prognosis for acute myeloid Leukemia (AML) is generally quite poor. The five-year survival rate for patients with AML is only around 27%. However, there are a number of factors that can affect a person's individual prognosis, including their age, overall health, and the specific subtype of AML they have. The survival rate for AML is notoriously low, but this is because it is a very aggressive form of cancer. The average life expectancy for people with AML is only around three to six months from the time of diagnosis. However, there are a small number of people who are able to achieve remission and live for many years after their diagnosis. There are a number of clinical trials currently underway that are exploring new treatment options for AML. These new treatments are showing promise and may improve the survival rate for this disease in the future. If you or someone you love has been diagnosed with AML, it is important to remember that there is hope. New treatments are being developed all the time and there is a chance that a cure for this disease will be found in the future. In the meantime, the best thing you can do is to stay positive and fight for every day.

What are the 3 stages of AML Leukemia?

The three stages of AML Leukemia are: Stage 1: In this stage, the Leukemia cells are growing quickly and crowding out the healthy blood cells in your bone marrow. This can cause problems with bleeding and infection. Stage 2: In this stage, the Leukemia cells have spread to other parts of your body, such as your lymph nodes, liver, or spleen. Stage 3: In this stage, the Leukemia cells have spread to your brain or spinal cord.

Is AML Leukemia curable?

When it comes to Leukemia, there are four main types that have been identified. These include: -acute lymphocytic Leukemia (ALL) -acute myelogenous Leukemia (AML) -chronic lymphocytic Leukemia (CLL) -chronic myelogenous Leukemia (CML) Of these, AML is the most common type of Leukemia in adults, accounting for around 70-80% of all cases. This type of Leukemia is characterized by the overproduction of myeloblasts, which are immature white blood cells. While there are treatments available for Leukemia, the disease is currently incurable. However, with early diagnosis and treatment, many patients are able to achieve remission and enjoy long, healthy lives. There are a number of factors that contribute to whether or not a patient will achieve remission, including the type of Leukemia they have, their age, and their overall health. In general, patients with ALL have a higher chance of achieving remission than those with AML. That being said, there have been significant advancements in the treatment of Leukemia in recent years, and more and more patients are now able to achieve remission and lead healthy lives. With the help of modern medicine, it is hopeful that one day Leukemia will be a curable disease.

How aggressive is AML Leukemia?

Acute myeloid Leukemia (AML) is an aggressive type of Leukemia that can progress quickly if it is not treated promptly. The average survival rate for people with AML is only about 24% following diagnosis, which means that it is one of the most aggressive forms of Leukemia. Treatment for AML can be effective, but it is typically very intensive and often comes with significant side effects. In some cases, such as when the Leukemia is in its early stages, a bone marrow transplant may be recommended as the best treatment option.

How long do AML patients live?

The average life expectancy for a person with AML is around 3-6 months. However, many people have been known to live for much longer, with some people surviving for years. The reason that AML is so difficult to treat is because it is a cancer of the blood cells, which are constantly being replenished. This means that even if treatment is successful in destroying the cancer cells, they can quickly return. There is currently no cure for AML, but treatment can prolong a person's life and improve their quality of life. radiation therapy and chemotherapy are the most common treatments for AML. Radiation therapy uses high-energy beams to destroy cancer cells. Chemotherapy uses drugs to kill cancer cells. These treatments can be very effective in the early stages of AML, but they become less effective as the disease progresses. There are many different types of chemotherapy drugs, and they are often used in combinations. The most common chemotherapy drugs used to treat AML are cytarabine, daunorubicin, and idarubicin. Cytarabine is the most effective chemotherapy drug for AML, but it can also cause the most side effects. These side effects can include hair loss, mouth sores, nausea, and vomiting. Daunorubicin and idarubicin are less likely to cause side effects, but they are not as effective as cytarabine. Targeted therapy is a newer type of treatment that is becoming more common in the treatment of AML. This type of therapy targets specific genes or proteins that are found in cancer cells. This allows the treatment to kill cancer cells without harming normal cells. One of the most common targeted therapies used to treat AML is trimetrexate. Trimetrexate is a chemotherapy drug that is targeted to the gene that is responsible for the production of a protein called thymidylate synthase. This protein is necessary for cancer cells to survive. stem cell transplant is another option for treatment, particularly for people who are unable to have radiation therapy or chemotherapy. A stem cell transplant is a procedure in which healthy stem cells are injected into the body to replace the cancerous blood cells. The stem cells can be donated by a relative or friend, or they can be taken from the person's own body. This procedure is very risky, and it is only an option for people who are in good health. Although there is no cure for AML, treatment can prolong a person's life and improve their quality of life. It is important to discuss all treatment options with a doctor to find the best option for each individual.

Does AML spread quickly?

In general, leukaemia does not spread quickly. However, there are some aggressive subtypes, such as acute myeloid leukaemia (AML), which can progress rapidly. According to the Leukaemia & Blood Cancer New Zealand, AML is the most common type of adult leukaemia, and can often be difficult to treat. There are several factors that can affect the rate at which AML progresses. For example, the cancer may be more aggressive in people who are younger, or who have certain genetic abnormalities. In some cases, the cancer can spread to other parts of the body, such as the brain or spine. Treatment for AML often involves a combination of chemotherapy and radiation therapy. In some cases, a bone marrow transplant may also be recommended. The goal of treatment is to kill the cancer cells and stop them from spreading. Although AML can be a very serious cancer, the prognosis has improved in recent years. With early diagnosis and aggressive treatment, many people with AML can achieve remission and go on to lead long and healthy lives.

What triggers AML Leukemia?

When it comes to cancer, there are a lot of different Triggering factors. In most cases, the body's ability to fight off cancer cells is lowered, either due to a weakened immune system, or due to changes in the DNA of the cells. However, in some cases, it's not entirely clear what causes cancer. In the case of acute myeloid Leukemia (AML), there are several possible triggers that could be responsible. The first potential trigger is radiation exposure. This could be from things like X-rays or other types of cancer treatments. In some cases, people who have been exposed to high levels of radiation are more likely to develop AML later on in life. Another potential trigger is chemicals. There are a lot of different chemicals that are used in industry and other settings, and some of them have been linked to cancer.

Benzene, for example, is a known carcinogen, and people who are exposed to it are at increased risk for developing AML. Some viruses have also been linked to AML. The most well-known is the human T-cell Leukemia virus (HTLV-1). This virus is most commonly found in Japan, the Caribbean, and parts of Africa, and people who are infected with it are at increased risk for developing AML. Finally, there are some genetic factors that can increase the risk for AML. For example, people with certain blood disorders, like polycythemia vera or essential thrombocythemia, are more likely to develop AML. Additionally, people who have certain genetic mutations, like the BRCA1 or BRCA2 mutations, are also at increased risk. AML is a complex disease, and there are most likely several different factors that contribute to its development. In most cases, it's not possible to identify a single trigger. However, understanding the potential triggers is important for developing better treatments and for prevention.

Leukaemia is a serious illness that can have a significant impact on a person's quality of life. It is important to be aware of the symptoms of leukaemia and to seek medical advice if you think you may have the condition. There is no one definitive treatment for leukaemia and the most appropriate treatment will be decided by a specialist based on the individual's circumstances. With the right treatment and support, many people with leukaemia can manage their condition and live long and fulfilling lives.

How quickly does AML progress?

The average person with leukaemia experiences a rapid onset of symptoms. In fact, the average time from diagnosis to death is just over three months. Of course, some people may experience a more prolonged battle with the disease, while others may succumb to it more quickly. In any case, leukaemia is generally a very aggressive disease. So, how quickly does AML progress? Unfortunately, there is no one-size-fits-all answer to this question. The rate at which leukaemia progresses can vary greatly from person to person. In some cases, the disease may progression quickly, while in others it may progress more slowly. There are a number of factors that can affect the rate at which leukaemia progresses. These include the type of leukaemia, the person's age, and the person's overall health. In general, however, leukaemia is a very aggressive disease that progresses quickly. That is why it is so important to get an early diagnosis and to start treatment as soon as possible.

What were your first AML symptoms?

I was diagnosed with leukaemia in 2013. I was 22 years old. I had been feeling tired for a few months and had started to get bruising on my arms and legs. I also had a fever and felt generally unwell. I went to my GP and had some blood tests. The results showed that I had a high white blood cell count and I was referred to a specialist. I had more blood tests and a bone marrow biopsy. The diagnosis was acute myeloid leukaemia. I was started on chemotherapy straight away. The first few months were really tough. I had a lot of side effects from the treatment and felt very unwell. I lost my hair and had to stay in hospital for long periods of time. It has now been six years since my diagnosis and I am doing well. I am in remission and have finished treatment. I am grateful to all the doctors and nurses who have helped me through my journey.

What are the 5 stages of Leukemia ML?

Acute myeloid Leukemia (AML) is a cancer of the blood and bone marrow. The bone marrow is the soft tissue inside your bones where your blood cells are made. AML is a type of cancer that affects the white blood cells. AML is considered to be a fast-growing cancer. There are five main stages of AML, though some doctors may further divide these stages into sub-stages. The stages are: Stage 0: In stage 0, abnormal white blood cells are found in the bone marrow, but they do not yet form cancer and they have not spread to any other parts of the body. Stage I: In stage I, abnormal white blood cells are found in the bone marrow and they have started to form cancer. The cancer has not yet spread to any other parts of the body. Stage II: In stage II, the cancer has spread from the bone marrow to the blood. The cancer may have also spread to other organs, such as the liver or the spleen. Stage III: In stage III, the cancer has spread from the bone marrow to the blood and to one or more organs. Stage IV: In stage IV, the cancer has spread from the bone marrow to the blood and to two or more organs.

Is AML considered terminal?

Acute myeloid Leukemia (AML) is considered to be a potentially terminal cancer. However, there are many different factors that contribute to prognosis, including the individual's age, general health, and the specific subtype of AML. In some cases, treatment may be able to cure the cancer, while in others, it may only be possible to manage the symptoms and prolong life. The overall five-year survival rate for AML is 26%, but this can vary widely based on individual factors. For example, the five-year survival rate is 64% for children and adolescents with AML, while it is only 14% for adults over the age of 60. In general, the survival rate is higher for those who are diagnosed at an earlier age and who have a healthier lifestyle. There are many different treatment options available for AML, including chemotherapy, radiation therapy, stem cell transplant, and targeted therapy. The specific treatment plan will be determined by the individual's age, health, and the specific subtype of AML. In some cases, multiple rounds of treatment may be necessary. AML is a serious cancer that can be fatal, but there are many different factors that contribute to prognosis. With advances in treatment options, there is hope for a cure for many people diagnosed with AML.

Does AML come on suddenly?

AML usually comes on suddenly, without any warning signs. This can be very frightening for patients and their families. The symptoms of AML can vary from person to person, and they may come and go over time. Some people with AML may have only a few symptoms, while others may have many. The most common symptoms of AML include: - Fatigue - Shortness of breath - easy bruising or bleeding - Fever - Weight loss - Pain in the bones or joints These symptoms can be caused by other conditions, so it is important to see a doctor if you are worried about them. AML is often diagnosed after a person has a blood test.

How long does chemo last for AML?

You might have chemotherapy for a few months or longer, depending on how well you respond to treatment. Chemotherapy for AML is usually given in cycles. Each cycle takes 4 to 7 weeks. You will have a week of treatment, followed by 3 weeks of rest. This is considered 1 cycle. Most people need at least 2 to 3 cycles of chemotherapy, and some people may need up to 6 cycles. If your cancer is in remission after the first few cycles of chemotherapy, your doctor may suggest that you have 1 more cycle of treatment to help prevent the cancer from coming back. If your cancer does not respond to chemotherapy, or if it comes back after treatment, you may be offered other types of treatment, such as a stem cell transplant.

Is AML Leukemia genetic?

Leukaemia is a cancer of the blood cells. The four main types of leukaemia are: - Acute lymphoblastic leukaemia (ALL) - Acute myeloid leukaemia (AML) - Chronic lymphocytic leukaemia (CLL) - Chronic myeloid leukaemia (CML) Blood cells are made in the bone marrow. In leukaemia, there is an overproduction of abnormal blood cells. These abnormal cells crowd out the healthy blood cells, causing problems with bleeding and infection. Leukaemia is usually treated with chemotherapy, which kills the cancerous cells. However, chemotherapy can also kill healthy cells, which can cause side-effects such as hair loss, nausea and fatigue. There are many different causes of leukaemia, including exposure to certain chemicals and radiation, as well as certain genetic conditions. However, the exact cause of leukaemia is often unknown. So, is AML Leukemia genetic? While the exact cause of AML is unknown, there are certain risk factors that may increase your chances of developing the disease. These include: - Exposure to certain chemicals or radiation - Certain genetic conditions - A family history of leukaemia While these risk factors may increase your chances of developing AML, it is important to remember that most people with these risk factors will never develop the disease. If you have been diagnosed with AML, it is important to work with your medical team to develop a treatment plan that is right for you.

A diagnosis of leukaemia is life-changing. It can be difficult to cope with the diagnosis and treatment can be intense. However, it is important to remember that treatment is often successful and there are many support options available. With the right treatment and support, many people with leukaemia go on to live long and healthy lives.

Who is most likely to get AML?

There are many different types of leukaemia, and the most common type is acute myeloid leukaemia (AML). AML is more common in adults than in children, and the average age of diagnosis is around 70. However, anyone can develop AML at any age. People with certain genetic disorders, such as Down syndrome, are at increased risk of developing AML. People who have been exposed to certain chemicals, such as benzene, are also at increased risk.Smoking cigarettes is also a risk factor for AML. People with certain blood disorders, such as myelodysplastic syndromes, are at increased risk of developing AML. People who have had certain types of cancer, such as Hodgkin's disease, are also at increased risk. There are many other risk factors for AML, including family history, certain infections, and certain medications. However, the exact cause of AML is unknown in most cases.

Can AML run in families?

In short, yes, AML can run in families. This is because cancer is largely a genetic disease, and AML is no exception. Families with a history of cancer are more likely to have members with AML. AML is a cancer of the blood and bone marrow. The bone marrow is where blood cells are made. In AML, the bone marrow makes abnormal white blood cells. These abnormal cells crowd out the healthy blood cells, making it hard for the blood to do its job. AML can be caused by a genetic mutation, which can be inherited from a parent. This is why families with a history of cancer are more likely to have members with AML. In some cases, the genetic mutation that causes AML may be spontaneous, meaning it is not inherited. If you have a family member with AML, you may be at an increased risk of developing the disease. If you are concerned about your risk, talk to your doctor. They can discuss your family history and whether you should be screened for AML.

What are the end stages of AML Leukemia?

The end stages of AML Leukemia are marked by the cancerous cells taking over the bone marrow and producing abnormal white blood cells. This can lead to a decrease in the number of healthy blood cells, including red blood cells and platelets. This can cause fatigue, easy bruising or bleeding, and an increased risk of infection. In some cases, the Leukemia cells may also spread to other organs, such as the liver or brain. Treatment for AML at this stage is typically more aggressive, and may include chemotherapy, stem cell transplant, or targeted therapy.

What organs are affected by AML?

Although acute myeloid leukaemia (AML) is classified according to which cells in the bone marrow are affected, the cancerous cells can also spread to other organs. The most common organs affected by AML are the liver and the spleen, where the cancerous cells can build up and cause the organs to enlarge. In some cases, the cancerous cells can also spread to the lungs, the brain, and the lymph nodes. The liver is one of the most common organs affected by AML. The cancerous cells can build up in the liver and cause it to enlarge. In some cases, the liver can become so enlarged that it can cause abdominal pain. In addition, the cancerous cells can also spread to the lungs and the brain. The spleen is another common organ affected by AML. The cancerous cells can build up in the spleen and cause it to enlarge. In some cases, the spleen can become so enlarged that it can cause abdominal pain. In addition, the cancerous cells can also spread to the lungs and the brain. The lungs are another common organ affected by AML. The cancerous cells can build up in the lungs and cause them to become enlarged. In some cases, the cancerous cells can also spread to the brain. The brain is another common organ affected by AML. The cancerous cells can build up in the brain and cause it to become enlarged. In some cases, the cancerous cells can also spread to the spinal cord. The lymph nodes are another common organ affected by AML. The cancerous cells can build up in the lymph nodes and cause them to become enlarged. In some cases, the cancerous cells can also spread to the lungs and the brain. In some cases, the cancerous cells can also spread to the bones. The cancerous cells can build up in the bones and cause them to become enlarged. In some cases, the cancerous cells can also spread to the spinal cord.

What is palliative care for AML?

Palliative care for AML is the care that focuses on providing relief from the symptoms, side effects, and stress of a serious illness. It is an important part of the overall care for AML patients and their families. The goal of palliative care is to improve the quality of life for both the patient and the family. Palliative care for AML can include many different services, such as help with pain and symptom management, emotional support, practical help, and spiritual care. Palliative care teams are made up of different specialists, including doctors, nurses, social workers, chaplains, and other professionals. Palliative care can be provided in the hospital, at home, or in other settings, such as hospices or palliative care units. Palliative care for AML is important because it can help to improve the quality of life for both the patient and the family. It can also help to relieve the symptoms and side effects of the disease. In some cases, palliative care can also help to prolong life.

How many rounds of chemo is needed for AML?

When it comes to Leukemia, specifically AML, there is no one size fits all answer to the question of how many rounds of chemo is needed. It varies depending on the individual and the severity of their case. In general, though, most people with AML will need to go through several rounds of chemotherapy in order to see any real results. The specific number will be determined by your doctor, but it is not uncommon for people to need 4-6 rounds of chemo before they start to see any significant improvements. While the chemotherapy is undoubtedly tough, it is important to remember that it is also the best chance for a cure. The majority of people who are diagnosed with AML will not be able to achieve remission without undergoing chemo. Even with the chemo, the chances of achieving a cure are not great, but they are still much better than if you were to receive no treatment at all. It is also worth noting that the number of rounds of chemo needed can change over the course of treatment. If the first few rounds do not seem to be working as well as hoped, your doctor may recommend additional rounds. Similarly, if the first few rounds are particularly effective, you may be able to finish treatment sooner than originally anticipated. No one deserves to have to go through Leukemia, but if you are diagnosed with AML, it is important to remember that chemotherapy is your best chance for a cure. It is not going to be easy, but it is worth it.

What is the 7 day rule in chemotherapy?

Cancer cells divide more rapidly than healthy cells, so chemotherapy drugs that target rapidly dividing cells are used to treat cancer. The 7 day rule is the standard for how often chemotherapy is given. This means that cancer patients will receive chemotherapy every 7 days. There are a few exceptions to the 7 day rule. For example, if a patient is receiving a very intense chemotherapy regimen, they may be given chemotherapy every 3-4 days. Some chemotherapy drugs can be given once a week. And some chemotherapy drugs are given as a continuous infusion, which means the patient will receive the drug through a needle or catheter 24 hours a day for several days or weeks. The 7 day rule is not set in stone, and may be different for each patient depending on the type of chemotherapy they are receiving. Your doctor will determine the schedule that is best for you.

The most common type of leukaemia is acute lymphoblastic leukaemia (ALL), which accounts for about 75% of all leukaemia cases diagnosed in children. It is also the most common type of cancer in children. The outlook for children with ALL has improved significantly over the past few decades, with cure rates now exceeding 80%.

Can you have AML for years and not know it?

Leukaemia is a cancer of the blood cells. It can affect any age group, but is most common in children and young adults. The four main types of leukaemia are acute lymphoblastic leukaemia (ALL), acute myeloid leukaemia (AML), chronic lymphocytic leukaemia (CLL) and chronic myeloid leukaemia (CML). ALL starts in the bone marrow (the spongy tissue inside the bones where blood cells are made) and grows quickly. AML also begins in the bone marrow, but grows more slowly. CLL starts in the lymphocytes (a type of white blood cell), and CML in the myeloid cells (another type of white blood cell). Leukaemia is treated with chemotherapy, which uses drugs to kill the cancer cells. In some cases, a stem cell transplant may be needed. This is where healthy stem cells (immature blood cells) are transplanted into the patient to replace the cancerous blood cells. Most people with leukaemia will have some symptoms, such as feeling tired, breathless, having a fever or bleeding more easily than normal. However, it is possible to have leukaemia for years without knowing it. This is because the symptoms can be mild, or may not appear until the cancer is at an advanced stage. If you have any concerns about your health, it is important to see your doctor for a check-up.

What is the survival rate for CLL Leukemia?

When it comes to cancer, there are many different types and subtypes – which can make treatment and predicting outcomes complicated. In chronic lymphocytic Leukemia (CLL), white blood cells called lymphocytes grow and multiply in an abnormal way. CLL is the most common type of Leukemia in adults, and while it can occur at any age, it is most often diagnosed in people over the age of 55. The American Cancer Society estimates that in 2020, there will be about 20,920 new cases of CLL in the United States. CLL treatment has improved dramatically in recent years. Thanks to new and better drugs, the average survival rate for CLL has increased from just over four years in the 1970s to nearly 11 years today. But while the average survival rate is encouraging, it doesn't tell the whole story. When it comes to cancer, survival rates are often expressed as a "five-year survival rate." This means that if 100 people are diagnosed with CLL, about 83 of them will still be alive five years later. But that doesn't mean that the other 17 people will have died from CLL. Some may have died from other causes, such as heart disease or another form of cancer. Others may still be alive but have stopped treatment because their cancer is in remission. The five-year survival rate for CLL has been slowly improving over the past few decades. In the 1970s, the five-year survival rate was just 24 percent. But by 2013, it had increased to 83 percent. Still, this means that about 17 percent of people with CLL will die from the disease within five years of their diagnosis. There are a number of factors that can affect a person's chances of surviving CLL. One of the most important is the stage of the disease. CLL is typically diagnosed in one of three stages: Stage I: The disease is limited to the lymph nodes. Stage II: The disease has spread to the spleen or liver. Stage III: The disease has spread to the bone marrow, blood, or other organs. People with stage I CLL have the best chance of surviving the disease. The five-year survival rate for stage I CLL is nearly 95 percent. But for people with stage III CLL, the five-year survival rate is only about 67 percent. Another important factor is the type of CLL. There are two main types of CLL: Type A: The disease progresses slowly and is less likely to require treatment. Type B: The disease progresses quickly and is more likely to require treatment. People with type A CLL have a better chance of surviving the disease than people with type B CLL. The five-year survival rate for type A CLL is about 90 percent. But for type B CLL, the five-year survival rate is only about

How serious is CLL cancer?

CLL is a cancer of the blood and bone marrow. The four main types of blood cancer are leukaemia, lymphoma, myeloma and thrombocytopenia. CLL is the most common type of leukaemia in the UK. CLL affects a type of white blood cell called a lymphocyte. Lymphocytes are part of the immune system and help to protect the body against infection. In CLL, the lymphocytes become abnormal and build up in the blood and bone marrow. The build-up of abnormal cells means that there are fewer healthy blood cells available to do their job. This can lead to anaemia (a reduction in the number of red blood cells), increased susceptibility to infections, and easy bruising or bleeding. CLL is usually a slow-growing cancer. It may not cause any symptoms for many years. When symptoms do occur, they are often generalised and non-specific, such as fatigue and weight loss. CLL is more common in older people, with the average age at diagnosis being 72. It is slightly more common in men than in women. CLL is usually diagnosed following a blood test. The doctor may also order a bone marrow biopsy (a procedure to remove a small sample of bone marrow for testing). CLL is treatable but not curable. The aim of treatment is to control the cancer and relieve symptoms. Treatment may not be necessary if the cancer is slow-growing and not causing any symptoms. Treatment options for CLL include chemotherapy, radiotherapy and targeted therapies. Stem cell transplantation may also be an option for some people. CLL is a serious cancer but it can be controlled with treatment. With advances in treatment, more and more people are living with CLL for many years.

How is CLL different from Leukemia?

The main difference between CLL and Leukemia is that CLL is a cancer of the blood that affects the white blood cells, whereas Leukemia is a cancer of the blood and bone marrow that affects both the white and red blood cells. CLL is much more common in adults over the age of 55, and the average age at diagnosis is 72. It is very rare in children. Leukemia is more common in children, but can occur at any age. CLL cells tend to build up in the blood over time and may not cause any symptoms for many years. When symptoms do occur, they may include fatigue, weight loss, night sweats, and easy bruising or bleeding. Leukemia cells can build up in the blood very quickly and may cause more severe symptoms such as fever, fatigue, weight loss, night sweats, easy bruising or bleeding, and pain or swelling in the abdomen or bones. CLL is usually treated with chemotherapy, and sometimes with targeted therapy or stem cell transplant. Leukemia is also treated with chemotherapy, but may also require radiation therapy or stem cell transplant.

Is CLL Leukemia fatal?

Leukemia is a type of cancer that starts in the blood cells. In most cases, Leukemia is not fatal. However, Chronic Lymphocytic Leukemia (CLL) is a type of Leukemia that is more aggressive and can be fatal. CLL is a cancer of the blood cells that starts in the bone marrow and then goes into the blood. It is the most common type of Leukemia in adults. CLL is more common in men than women. It is also more common in people of European descent. CLL is a slow-growing cancer. It can take years for it to get to a point where it is fatal. Treatment for CLL can keep the cancer from progressing and people can live for many years with the disease.

Can CLL patients live 20 years?

The average life expectancy for people with CLL is about 10 years. However, some people can live much longer – even 20 years or more. While there is no cure for CLL, treatments are becoming more effective, and many people with CLL now enjoy a good quality of life. Not everyone with CLL lives for 20 years, but it is becoming more common for people to reach this age. Some people with CLL die from unrelated causes, such as heart disease or stroke. Others may die from complications of CLL, such as infections. However, more and more people with CLL are surviving for 20 years or more. This is thanks to advances in treatment, which are making the disease more manageable. There are now a range of effective treatments available, including targeted therapies and immunotherapies. These treatments can help to control the disease and extend life expectancy. CLL is a slowly progressing disease, and many people with CLL live for many years without needing treatment. In some cases, treatment may not be necessary until the disease progresses. This means that people with CLL can often live relatively normal lives. If you have CLL, it is important to remember that you are not alone. There are many people in the world living with CLL, and treatments are becoming more and more effective. With the right treatment, it is possible to live for 20 years or more.

What should be avoided in CLL?

There are a few things that should be avoided if you have CLL. First, avoid drinking alcohol. It can interact with the medications used to treat CLL and make them less effective. Additionally, alcohol can also worsen some of the symptoms associated with CLL. Secondly, avoid smoking cigarettes. Cigarette smoke contains harmful chemicals that can damage the lungs and make it more difficult for the body to fight off infections. Additionally, smoking can also interfere with the effectiveness of CLL treatments. Finally, avoid contact with people who have infections. It is important to try to avoid exposure to viruses and bacteria as much as possible. People with

CLL are at an increased risk of developing serious infections. If you must be around someone who is sick, be sure to wash your hands frequently and avoid sharing personal items.

In conclusion, leukaemia is a serious illness that can have a devastating effect on patients and their families. However, with early diagnosis and treatment, many people with leukaemia can go on to lead long and healthy lives.

What age group is CLL most common?

Chronic lymphocytic leukaemia (CLL) is a type of leukaemia that most often affects older people. It is the most common type of leukaemia in people over the age of 55. In the UK, CLL is the second most common type of leukaemia after acute myeloid leukaemia (AML). CLL usually develops slowly over a number of years and, for many people, does not cause any problems. Some people with CLL may need treatment to control the symptoms and help keep them healthy. The cause of CLL is not known. It is not contagious and cannot be passed on to other people.

How quickly does CLL progress?

Cancer of the blood is often called Leukemia. It starts in the bone marrow, where blood cells are made. The bone marrow is the spongy tissue inside your bones. Leukemia usually starts in the white blood cells, which fight infection. But it can also occur in red blood cells, which carry oxygen to the body's tissues, or in platelets, which help the blood to clot. In most cases of Leukemia, the cancer cells build up slowly over months or years. But in some cases, the cells can multiply quickly. If the Leukemia is not treated, it can progress to a life-threatening illness. The rate at which Leukemia progresses can vary a great deal from one person to another. There are four main types of Leukemia, which are classified according to how quickly the disease progresses and the type of cells affected. • Acute lymphoblastic Leukemia (ALL) is the most common type of Leukemia in children. It can also occur in adults, but this is much less common. ALL progresses quickly and needs to be treated urgently. • Acute myeloid Leukemia (AML) is the most common type of Leukemia in adults. It progresses quickly and needs to be treated urgently. • Chronic lymphocytic Leukemia (CLL) progresses slowly and may not need to be treated immediately. • Chronic myeloid Leukemia (CML) progresses slowly and may not need to be treated immediately.

What is end stage CLL like?

Cancerous cells in the bone marrow crowd out the healthy blood cells, leading to a host of problems. A person with End Stage Chronic Lymphocytic Leukemia (CLL) may experience: -Anemia: This is a condition in which there are not enough healthy red blood cells to carry oxygen throughout the body. Anemia can cause fatigue, paleness, and shortness of breath. -Bleeding problems: A shortage of platelets (cell fragments that help with blood clotting) can cause excessive bleeding or bruising. -Infections: A shortage of white blood cells leaves the body vulnerable to infection. Even a minor infection can be serious for someone with CLL. -Swollen lymph nodes: Enlarged lymph nodes can cause pain and discomfort. They can also press on organs and cause other problems. -Fatigue: This is a common symptom of CLL, and can be caused by the cancer, the treatments, or anemia. -Weight loss: This can be caused by the cancer or the treatments. -Fever: This can be a symptom of infection or cancer. End Stage Chronic Lymphocytic Leukemia is a serious, life-threatening illness. With treatment, some people are able to live for many years. However, the disease will eventually progress and is ultimately fatal.

What is the 1st line treatment for CLL?

As with most cancers, treatment for CLL will vary depending on the individual case and the stage at which the cancer is diagnosed. The first line of treatment for CLL is typically chemotherapy. This may be given as a "cocktail" of different drugs, or as a targeted therapy aimed at the specific genetic changes that are found in the patient's cancer cells. For patients who are unsuitable for or do not respond to chemotherapy, other treatment options may be considered. These include targeted therapies such as monoclonal antibody therapy, radiation therapy and stem cell transplantation. The aim of treatment for CLL is to control the cancer and allow the patient to live as normal a life as possible. In some cases, this may mean simply managing the disease with regular monitoring and no active treatment. In other cases, treatment may be required to keep the cancer under control and help relieve any symptoms that the patient is experiencing.

How painful is CLL?

Cancer pain is unique and complex. It can be caused by the cancer itself, by treatments, or by other conditions that are unrelated to cancer. CLL pain is often caused by the cancer pressing on bones or nerves. The pain can vary from mild to severe and can be constant or come and go. Treatment can help to lessen the pain, but it is often difficult to control. Cancer pain can be caused by the cancer itself, by treatments, or by other conditions that are unrelated to cancer. CLL pain is often caused by the cancer pressing on bones or nerves. The pain can vary from mild to severe and can be constant or come and go. Treatment can help to lessen the pain, but it is often difficult to control. Cancer pain is unique and complex. It can vary widely in intensity, duration, and quality. It can be sharp or dull, constant or intermittent. Cancer pain can be caused by the cancer itself, by treatments, or by other conditions that are unrelated to cancer. CLL pain is often caused by the cancer pressing on bones or nerves. The pain can vary from mild to severe and can be constant or come and go. Treatment can help to lessen the pain, but it is often difficult to control. Cancer pain is unique and complex. It can vary widely in intensity, duration, and quality. It can be sharp or dull, constant or intermittent. Cancer pain can be caused by the cancer itself, by treatments, or by other conditions that are unrelated to cancer. CLL is a type of cancer that starts in the white blood cells. The main symptom of CLL is pain, caused by the cancer pressing on bones or nerves. The pain can vary from mild to severe and can be constant or come and go. Treatment can help to lessen the pain, but it is often difficult to control.

Does CLL shorten life expectancy?

CLL is the most common type of leukaemia in the Western world, and the average age of diagnosis is between 70 and 80 years old. The prognosis for patients with CLL has improved dramatically over the past few decades, and the majority of patients now survive for 10 or more years after diagnosis. However, the disease is still considered to be incurable, and the average life expectancy for patients with CLL is around 10-12 years. There are a number of factors that can affect the life expectancy of a patient with CLL, including the stage of the disease, the patient's age, and the presence of other health conditions. The stage of the disease is one of the most important prognostic factors in CLL. Patients who are diagnosed at an early stage of the disease (e.g. stage I or II) have a better prognosis than those who are diagnosed at a later stage (e.g. stage III or IV). Age is another important factor. Patients who are younger than 60 years old at the time of diagnosis tend to have a better prognosis than those who are older than 60 years old. The presence of other health conditions can also affect the life expectancy of a patient with CLL. For example, patients who have comorbidities such as diabetes or heart disease tend to have a shorter life expectancy than those who do not have these conditions. In general, the life expectancy of a patient with CLL is shorter than that of the general population. However, there is a wide range of individual prognoses, and some patients with CLL live for many years after diagnosis.

How do you know what stage you are with CLL?

The main way your doctor tells how advanced your CLL is, is by looking at the number of abnormal blood cells in your sample. The percentage of abnormal cells is called the blast count. If you have less than 5% blasts in your blood, it's called chronic lymphocytic leukaemia (CLL). If you have more than 5% blasts, it's called acute lymphoblastic leukaemia (ALL). CLL is further divided into stages, depending on the number of abnormal cells in your blood and bone marrow, and how much the disease has spread. There are 4 main stages of CLL: Stage 0: you have less than 5% abnormal cells in your blood. Stage 1: you have between 5-10% abnormal cells in your blood. Stage 2: you have between 11-20% abnormal cells in your blood. Stage 3: you have more than 20% abnormal cells in your blood. The higher the stage, the more advanced the disease. CLL doesn't usually cause any symptoms in the early stages. As the disease gets worse, you may start to feel fatigued and have a poor appetite. You may also get infections more easily. If you have CLL, your doctor will probably do blood tests every few months to check your blood cell counts. They may also do bone marrow tests to check the percentage ofblast cells.

The writer concludes by saying that leukaemia is not curable, but with new treatments and therapies, people with leukaemia can now live long and productive lives.

Does exercise help CLL?

Leukaemia is a cancer of the blood. It is a difficult disease to treat, and there is currently no cure. However, scientists are constantly working to find new ways to improve treatment and increase survival rates. Exercise has been shown to be beneficial for a range of health conditions, including cancer. Some studies have suggested that exercise may help to improve survival rates in people with leukaemia. One study looked at the effect of exercise on survival rates in people with chronic lymphocytic leukaemia (CLL). The study found that people who exercised regularly had a significantly lower risk of dying from the disease. another study, scientists looked at the effect of exercise on patients with acute myeloid leukaemia (AML). The study found that people who exercised regularly had a lower risk of the disease progressing and a higher survival rate. Exercise is thought to be beneficial for people with leukaemia for a number of reasons. Exercise can help to improve the function of the immune system, which is important in fighting the disease. Exercise also helps to reduce stress and improve wellbeing, both of which can help improve the course of the disease. If you are considering starting to exercise, it is important to speak to your doctor first. They will be able to advise you on the best type of exercise for you and how to stay safe while doing it.

What is the 15 year survival rate for CLL?

In the United States, the 15-year survival rate for chronic lymphocytic Leukemia (CLL) is approximately 83%. CLL is the most common type of Leukemia in adults, and the survival rate has been increasing in recent years, thanks to advances in treatment. CLL is a type of cancer that starts in the white blood cells. The cancerous cells build up in the bone marrow and lymph nodes, crowding out the healthy blood cells. This can lead to problems such as infections, anemia, and bleeding. There is no one "right" treatment for CLL, as the best approach depends on individual factors such as the person's age and health, the stage of the cancer, and the person's preferences. Some people with CLL may need treatment right away, while others may be able to wait and watch for the cancer to progress. Common treatments for CLL include chemotherapy, targeted therapy, and immunotherapy. Chemo uses drugs to kill cancer cells, while targeted therapy targets specific molecules involved in cancer cell growth. Immunotherapy uses the body's immune system to fight cancer. In some cases, a stem cell transplant may be an option. This treatment is usually only considered for people with aggressive forms of CLL or who have not responded to other treatments. The survival rate for CLL has been increasing in recent years, thanks to advances in treatment. With the right treatment, many people with CLL can live long and healthy lives.

What can trigger CLL?

Cancer of the blood cells, called leukaemia, can happen when the body produces too many abnormal blood cells. The three main types of leukaemia are acute lymphoblastic leukaemia (ALL), acute myeloid leukaemia (AML) and chronic lymphocytic leukaemia (CLL). CLL is the most common type of leukaemia in adults. Leukaemia can be caused by exposure to certain chemicals or radiation, by certain viruses, or by a combination of these factors. People with certain genetic disorders, such as Down syndrome, are also at increased risk. There are many different triggers that can cause CLL, with some still unknown. However, some possible triggers include: -Exposure to certain chemicals: Benzene is a chemical that is found in petrol and is used in the manufacture of plastics, resins and detergents. Exposure to high levels of benzene can increase the risk of developing CLL. -Exposure to radiation: Radiation therapy is used to treat cancer, but can also increase the risk of developing leukaemia. -Certain viruses: There is evidence that the Epstein-Barr virus, which is associated with the development of mononucleosis, can also increase the risk of CLL. -Certain genetic disorders: People with certain genetic disorders, such as

Down syndrome, are at increased risk of developing CLL. While the causes of CLL are still being investigated, there are certain risk factors that have been identified. These include exposure to certain chemicals and radiation, certain viral infections, and certain genetic disorders. However, further research is needed to confirm the role of these factors in the development of CLL.

What organs are affected by CLL?

Cancer of the blood is referred to as Leukemia. Chronic lymphocytic Leukemia (CLL) is the most common type of Leukemia in the Western world. It is a slow-growing cancer of a type of white blood cell called a lymphocyte. Lymphocytes are important for fighting infection, but in CLL they build up in the blood and bone marrow, crowding out healthy blood cells. The main organs affected by CLL are the blood and bone marrow. The bone marrow is the spongy tissue inside the bones where blood cells are made. In CLL, the bone marrow produces too many abnormal lymphocytes. These abnormal cells crowd out the healthy blood cells, including the red blood cells that carry oxygen around the body, and the platelets that help to stop bleeding. This can lead to fatigue, breathlessness, increased risk of infections, and easy bruising or bleeding. CLL can also affect the lymph nodes. The lymph nodes are small, bean-shaped glands found throughout the body. They are an important part of the lymphatic system, which is involved in fighting infection. In CLL, the lymph nodes may become enlarged and swollen. This can cause pain and discomfort, and can make it difficult to breathe or swallow. The spleen is another organ that can be affected by CLL. The spleen is located in the abdomen, just below the ribs on the left side. It is part of the lymphatic system and helps to filter out old and damaged blood cells. In CLL, the spleen may become enlarged and overloaded with abnormal lymphocytes. This can cause pain and discomfort, and can lead to a decreased production of healthy blood cells. CLL can also affect the liver. The liver is located in the abdomen, on the right side, just below the ribs. It is responsible for a range of important functions, including filtering the blood and producing bile. In CLL, the liver may become overwhelmed with abnormal lymphocytes. This can cause a build-up of toxins in the blood and can lead to liver damage. In severe cases, CLL can affect the central nervous system, including the brain and spinal cord. This can cause a range of symptoms, such as headaches, seizures, and problems with vision, balance, and coordination. CLL is a slow-growing cancer, and many people with CLL live for many years with the condition. However, it is a serious illness, and it can be fatal if it is not treated.

What is the 10 year survival rate for CLL?

Cll is the most common type of Leukemia in the united states. The average age of diagnosis is 72. The median 10-year survival rate for cll is 83%. The 5-year survival rate is 64%. The 1-year survival rate is 47%. The prognosis for cll is generally good, with the majority of people surviving for many years after diagnosis. There are treatments available that can help prolong life and improve quality of life for people with cll.

What is very high risk CLL?

CLL is the most common type of leukaemia in adults and usually starts to develop later in life. It is a cancer of the blood cells that usually occurs in the white blood cells. The abnormal blood cells produced by CLL crowd out the healthy blood cells, which can lead to serious health problems. There are different types of CLL, each with its own prognosis. Some forms of CLL are more aggressive than others and can progress quickly, while other forms are slower-growing and may not need treatment for many years. very high risk CLL is a form of the disease that is more aggressive and progresses quickly. People with very high risk CLL have a higher chance of the disease getting worse and may need to start treatment sooner.

Does CLL go to the brain?

Leukaemia is a cancer of the blood cells. The four main types of leukaemia are lymphocytic, myeloid, acute and chronic. Lymphocytic leukaemia is the most common type of leukaemia in adults and accounts for about 30% of all leukaemia cases. Lymphocytic leukaemia starts in the lymphocytes, which are a type of white blood cell. Lymphocytes are made in the bone marrow and help to fight infection. Myeloid leukaemia is the second most common type of leukaemia in adults and accounts for about 25% of all leukaemia cases. Myeloid leukaemia starts in the myeloid cells, which are a type of white blood cell. Myeloid cells are made in the bone marrow and help to fight infection. Acute leukaemia is the most common type of leukaemia in children and accounts for about 40% of all leukaemia cases. Acute leukaemia starts in the lymphocytes, which are a type of white blood cell. Lymphocytes are made in the bone marrow and help to fight infection. Chronic leukaemia is the most common type of leukaemia in adults and accounts for about 30% of all leukaemia cases. Chronic leukaemia starts in the myeloid cells, which are a type of white blood cell. Myeloid cells are made in the bone marrow and help to fight infection. Leukaemia can spread to different parts of the body, including the brain. However, it is not clear how common this is. A study in the United States found that 2.3% of people with leukaemia had brain involvement at the time of diagnosis. There are different types of brain involvement in leukaemia. The most common type is leukaemic meningitis, which is when the leukaemia cells spread to the lining of the brain and spinal cord. Leukaemic meningitis is more common in children than adults. The second type of brain involvement is leukaemic encephalopathy, which is when the leukaemia cells spread to the brain tissue. Leukaemic encephalopathy is more common in adults than children. The third type of brain involvement is leukaemic brain tumours, which are rare. Leukaemic brain tumours are more common in children than adults. The treatment for leukaemia that has spread to the brain is the same as the treatment for leukaemia that has not spread to the brain. The main treatment for leukaemia is chemotherapy. Chemotherapy can be given as tablets, injection or infusion. If you have leukaemia and it has spread to your brain, it is important to be treated by a team of specialists who are experienced in treating leukaemia that has spread to the brain.

Leukaemia is a potentially fatal disease that can affect people of all ages. Early diagnosis and treatment is essential for the best possible outcome. With advances in medical care, more people are now able to receive the treatment they need and go on to lead long and healthy lives.

Can CLL spread to other organs?

Can CLL spread to other organs? Chronic lymphocytic Leukemia (CLL) is a type of cancer that starts from white blood cells in the bone marrow. The cancerous cells then spread into the blood. In most cases, CLL will not cause any symptoms and can go undetected for many years. However, as the cancer progresses, it may start to affect other organs in the body. The spread of CLL from the blood into other organs is known as metastasis. Metastasis usually occurs when the cancer has spread from the blood into the lymph nodes. However, it is also possible for CLL to spread to other organs such as the liver, lungs, and brain. The chances of metastasis depend on a number of factors, such as the stage of the cancer, the type of CLL, and the patient's age. In general, younger patients with early-stage CLL are less likely to experience metastasis than older patients with late-stage CLL. Treatment for CLL can often help to control the cancer and prolong the patient's life. However, there is no cure for CLL and it is not yet known how to prevent the cancer from spreading to other organs. If you have CLL, it is important to talk to your doctor about the risks of metastasis and the available treatment options.

What is the survival rate of Leukemia CML?

The average age of a person at diagnosis with CML is 64 years. The median age of death from CML is 71 years. The 5-year overall survival rate from CML is 65%. The 10-year overall survival rate from CML is 53%. The 15-year overall survival rate from CML is 42%. CML is a type of Leukemia that progresses slowly compared to other types of Leukemia. The median survival time from CML is 10 years or more. The 5-year overall survival rate from CML is 65%. The 10-year overall survival rate from CML is 53%. The 15-year overall survival rate from CML is 42%. CML is a cancer of the blood and bone marrow. The vast majority of people with CML are diagnosed in the chronic phase, which is the least advanced phase of the disease. In the chronic phase, most people with CML have a good prognosis and a normal life expectancy. The median age of death from CML is 71 years. However, with advances in treatment, more and more people are living longer with CML. The 5-year overall survival rate from CML is 65%. The 10-year overall survival rate from CML is 53%. The 15-year overall survival rate from CML is 42%. CML is treatable but not curable. The first line of treatment for CML is a targeted therapy called imatinib (Gleevec). Imatinib works by targeting and inhibiting the Bcr-Abl protein, which is abnormal in people with CML. Imatinib is very effective in the chronic phase of CML. The majority of people who take imatinib will achieve a complete cytogenetic response, meaning that the treatments shrinks the number of abnormal cells in the blood. Although there is no cure for CML, treatment can control the disease and people can live for many years with a good quality of life. The 5-year overall survival rate from

CML is 65%. The 10-year overall survival rate from CML is 53%. The 15-year overall survival rate from CML is 42%.

Is CML life threatening?

Chronic myeloid leukaemia (CML) is a cancer of the blood and bone marrow. It is a type of leukaemia that progresses slowly and can be treated with medication. In some cases, CML can be cured with a bone marrow transplant. CML is caused by a genetic mutation that produces an abnormal protein called BCR-ABL. This protein causes the bone marrow to produce too many white blood cells. The excess white blood cells crowd out the healthy blood cells in the marrow and circulate in the blood. CML is a chronic disease, which means it can last for months or years. It is usually diagnosed in people over the age of 55. However, it is possible for people of any age to develop CML. CML is treated with medication that targets the BCR-ABL protein. This type of medication is called a tyrosine kinase inhibitor (TKI). TKIs work by blocking the activity of the BCR-ABL protein. This slows down the production of white blood cells and helps to keep the disease under control. In some cases, a bone marrow transplant may be recommended. This is a treatment that replaces the diseased bone marrow with healthy bone marrow from a donor. A bone marrow transplant can cure CML. CML is a serious disease, but it is not life-threatening. With treatment, most people with CML can live for many years.

Is CML a good cancer?

CML is a type of blood cancer that is relatively rare, accounting for only about 1% of all Leukemias. People with CML often have a good prognosis and a high survival rate. In fact, the overall five-year survival rate for CML is approximately 85%. While CML is certainly not a good cancer, it is not as aggressive as some other types of Leukemia. CML is typically diagnosed in adults over the age of 55, however, it can occur at any age. The average age at diagnosis is 65. The majority of CML cases are diagnosed in men. Caucasian men are more likely to develop CML than any other demographic. There are a few risk factors for CML, though the cause is unknown in most cases. Having a family member with CML increases one's risk. People with certain genetic disorders, such as Down syndrome, are also more likely to develop CML. People who have been exposed to certain chemicals, such as benzene, are also at increased risk. CML is a slow-growing cancer that starts in the bone marrow. The bone marrow is the soft tissue inside the bones where blood cells are made. In CML, the bone marrow produces too many white blood cells. The excess white blood cells crowd out the healthy blood cells, which can lead to a host of problems. People with CML may not have any symptoms in the early stages of the disease. When symptoms do appear, they may include fatigue, weakness, shortness of breath, and weight loss. As the disease progresses, people may experience bleeding and bruising, bone pain, and enlargement of the spleen. CML is typically treated with targeted therapy. Targeted therapy is a type of cancer treatment that targets specific genes, proteins, or the tissue environment that contributes to cancer growth and survival. This type of therapy is usually more effective and has fewer side effects than traditional chemotherapy. There are a few different targeted therapies used to treat CML. Imatinib (Gleevec) is the most common targeted therapy used. It works by inhibiting a protein that is necessary for cancer cell growth. Dasatinib (Sprycel) and nilotinib (Tasigna) are other targeted therapies that work in a similar way. Targeted therapy is usually very effective in treating CML. In most cases, the cancer is controlled with targeted therapy and people are able to live relatively normal lives. In some cases, the cancer may eventually become resistant to targeted therapy. When this happens, other treatment options, such as stem cell transplant, may be used. While CML is not a good cancer, it is not as aggressive as some other types of Leukemia and most people have a good prognosis. With targeted therapy, the cancer is usually controlled and people are able to live relatively normal lives.

How do you get CML Leukemia?

Leukaemia is a type of cancer that starts in the blood cells. The blood cells are made in the bone marrow, which is the spongy tissue inside the bones. In people with leukaemia, the bone marrow produces abnormal blood cells. The abnormal cells are Leukemia cells. They do not function properly and crowd out the normal blood cells. Leukemia cells can build up in the blood and bone marrow, and they can spread to other parts of the body, such as the lymph nodes, liver, brain, and spinal cord. When this happens, it is called advanced leukaemia. Leukaemia is usually divided into four main types, based on how quickly the disease develops and what kind of blood cells are affected. The most common type of leukaemia in adults is chronic myeloid leukaemia (CML). In CML, the abnormal cells are mostly myeloid cells. Myeloid cells turn into red blood cells, platelets, and some types of white blood cells. CML is a slow-growing form of leukaemia. In the early stages of CML, people may not have any symptoms. As the disease gets worse, people may have fatigue, weight loss, and fever. In the advanced stages, people may have bleeding and infection. CML is caused by a genetic change in the myeloid cells. The exact cause of this change is not known. However, it is not caused by anything you have done or anything you have been exposed to. CML is treated with medication. The goal of treatment is to control the disease and reduce the number of abnormal cells in the blood and bone marrow.

How long can a CML patient live?

There is no one definitive answer to how long a CML patient can live. CML is a chronic blood cancer, which means that it progresses slowly and can often be controlled with treatment. In general, the prognosis for CML patients has improved significantly in recent years. The average life expectancy for CML patients has increased from around 3-5 years in the 1970s to around 10-15 years in the 1980s and 1990s. However, there are a number of factors that can affect a person's prognosis, such as their age, their overall health, and the type of treatment they receive. In general, CML patients who are younger and in good health have a better prognosis than those who are older or have other health problems. The type of treatment a patient receives can also affect their prognosis. For example, patients who receive targeted therapy drugs such as imatinib (Gleevec) have a better prognosis than those who receive traditional chemotherapy. The specific characteristics of a person's CML can also affect their prognosis. For example, patients with a particular genetic mutation known as the Philadelphia chromosome have a worse prognosis than those without this mutation. As research into CML continues, it is hoped that the prognosis for CML patients will continue to improve. There are a number of new treatments under development that show promise in treating the disease. With continued improvements in treatment, it is possible that the life expectancy for CML patients will continue to increase in the years to come.

Is CML treated with chemo?

In general, CML is considered to be a treatable cancer with a good prognosis. The standard treatment for CML is targeted therapy with drugs that selectively target specific mutated proteins that are found only in cancer cells. These targeted drugs are typically very effective at slowing down the progression of CML and often result in long-term remission. Although targeted therapy is the standard treatment for CML, some people may also require chemotherapy if their CML is resistant to targeted therapy or if they have a severe reaction to the targeted therapy drugs. Chemotherapy is typically used as a last resort treatment option for CML, as it can have a number of serious side effects.

Leukaemia is a cancer of the blood cells. It is the most common type of cancer in children, but can also affect adults. Treatment for leukaemia can be complex and expensive, but many people can be successfully treated and cured.

What are the signs of CML getting worse?

As Leukemia cells develop and multiply, they crowd out healthy blood cells in the bone marrow. This makes it harder for the healthy blood cells to do their jobs. Crowding also can lead to low blood counts, which can cause a number of problems, such as: Anemia. Low red blood cell counts can cause tiredness, weakness and shortness of breath. Bleeding. Low platelet counts can cause easy bruising, bleeding gums and nosebleeds. Infections. Low white blood cell counts can increase the risk for infections. As the Leukemia cells continue to expand in the bone marrow, they begin to spill into the blood. In some cases, the Leukemia cells can also settle in other parts of the body, such as the liver, lungs, brain or spinal cord. These changes can cause a number of new symptoms, such as: Fever Weight loss Bone and joint pain Swollen lymph nodes Headaches If you are experiencing any of these symptoms, it is important to contact your doctor so that they can determine the cause and provide you with the appropriate treatment.

What organs are affected by CML?

CML, or Chronic Myeloid Leukaemia, is a cancer of the blood and bone marrow. The bone marrow is the soft, spongy tissue inside the bones where blood cells are made. In CML, the bone marrow produces too many immature white blood cells, called blasts. The blasts crowd out the healthy blood cells, making it harder for the blood to do its job. CML affects mostly adults over the age of 55, although it can occasionally occur in younger adults and children. There is no known cause of CML, although it is believed to be caused by a change, or mutation, in a gene. CML is not contagious and cannot be passed from one person to another. Treatment for CML usually begins with medication, which can help to control the number of blasts in the blood and bone marrow and improve the patient's symptoms. In some cases, a stem cell transplant may be recommended. This is a procedure in which the patient's own stem cells, or those from a donor, are transplanted into the patient to replace the damaged bone marrow.

What is the best treatment for CML?

chronic myelogenous Leukemia (CML), is a type of cancer that starts in the blood-forming cells of the bone marrow. The cancerous cells then invade the blood. As the cancer cells build up in the blood, they crowd out the healthy blood cells. This can lead to a low number of healthy red blood cells, white blood cells, and platelets. CML is treated with targeted therapy. Targeted therapy is a type of cancer treatment that uses drugs or other substances to identify and attack specific cancer cells without harming normal cells. The two main types of targeted therapy used to treat CML are tyrosine kinase inhibitors (TKIs) and immunotherapy. TKIs are the most common type of targeted therapy used to treat CML. They work by blocking the activity of a protein called BCR-ABL. This protein is made by the cancerous cells in CML and is needed for the cancer cells to grow. TKIs can effectively stop the growth of cancer cells and may even shrink the tumors. Immunotherapy is another type of targeted therapy that can be used to treat CML. It works by boosting the immune system's ability to fight cancer. Immunotherapy can be used in conjunction with TKIs or as a standalone treatment. The best treatment for CML depends on the individual patient. Some patients may respond well to TKIs alone, while others may require immunotherapy in addition to TKIs. The decision on which treatment to use is made by the patient's doctor, taking into account the patient's specific situation.

What were your first CML symptoms?

The first CML symptoms I remember were feeling really tired all the time, and just not having any energy. I would get out of breath really easily, and just generally felt really unwell. I also started to get bruising and bleeds more easily, and my spleen started to get enlarged. I went to my GP and they did some blood tests and that's when they found out I had leukaemia.

What is the first stage of CML?

The first stage of chronic myeloid Leukemia (CML) is the chronic phase. This phase can last for many years and usually has a good prognosis. In the chronic phase, the cancer is still growing, but it is slower than in the earlier, more aggressive stages. During the chronic phase, patients may have no symptoms or only mild symptoms. They may feel tired and have a loss of appetite, but they can usually still function normally. Some patients may need treatment to relieve symptoms or to reduce the risk of the disease progressing to a more serious stage. The chronic phase of CML is often treated with medication, such as tyrosine kinase inhibitors (TKIs). These drugs work by targeting the cancer cells and stopping them from growing. TKIs can be very effective at treating the chronic phase of CML, and they often allow patients to live long and healthy lives.

Is CML considered a rare disease?

CML, or Chronic Myelogenous Leukemia, is a slowly progressing cancer of the blood and bone marrow. In the United States, CML affects about 6,000 adults each year. Although the Leukemia can occur at any age, most people are diagnosed when they are 65 or older. CML is considered a rare disease. The term "rare disease" is used to describe a wide range of disorders that affect a small percentage of the population. In the United States, a rare disease is defined as a condition that affects fewer than 200,000 people. CML meets this definition and is therefore considered a rare disease. Although CML is considered rare, it is actually one of the more common forms of Leukemia. There are four main types of Leukemia, and CML is the second most common type of adult Leukemia, after acute lymphocytic Leukemia (ALL). CML is also the most common type of chronic Leukemia in adults. Despite its classification as a rare disease, CML is actually not that rare. In the United States, the condition affects about 6,000 adults each year. However, because CML is a slow-progressing cancer, many people live for years without knowing they have the disease. It is estimated that there are more than 100,000 people living with CML in the United States. CML is a treatable disease. In the past, the only treatment option for CML was a bone marrow transplant. However, there have been major advances in treatment in recent years. The FDA has approved two targeted therapies for CML, imatinib (Gleevec) and dasatinib (Sprycel). These drugs are effective in treating the disease and allowing people to live normal, healthy lives. Although CML is considered a rare disease, it is actually fairly common. There are treatments available that can help people live normal, healthy lives. If you think you may have CML, talk to your doctor.

How long is chemotherapy for CML?

There are many different types of chemotherapy, and the specific one that is used to treat CML can vary depending on the individual case. However, most courses of chemotherapy for CML last around 3 to 6 months. The reason that chemotherapy can take such a long time is because CML is a very slowly progressing disease. Even though chemotherapy is very effective at treating CML, it can take months or even years for the treatment to have its full effect. This is why it is so important for people with CML to be monitored closely by their medical team during and after treatment. One of the most important things to remember about chemotherapy is that it is not a cure. Even though it can effectively treat CML, the disease can still come back after treatment has finished. This is why it is so important for people with CML to stay on top of their health and to see their doctor regularly for check-ups.

Although leukaemia is a serious form of blood cancer, it is treatable and many people with leukaemia go on to live long and healthy lives. With advances in medical technology, the outlook for people with leukaemia is improving all the time. If you or someone you know has been diagnosed with leukaemia, there is no need to despair – there is help out there.

Can CML turn into other cancers?

There are many types of Leukemia, and chronic myeloid Leukemia (CML) is just one of them. CML is a type of cancer that starts in the bone marrow, where blood cells are made. In CML, the bone marrow makes too many white blood cells. These extra white blood cells are not able to fight infection very well, so people with CML are at an increased risk for infection. CML can be a very slow-growing cancer, and some people with CML may never need treatment. However, for other people, CML can grow quickly and may require treatment. Treatment for CML usually involves taking medication to kill the cancer cells. CML is considered to be a chronic cancer, which means it can last for a long time. In some cases, people with CML can live for many years with the disease. However, CML can also progress to other types of Leukemia, which can be more difficult to treat. So, can CML turn into other cancers? While CML can progress to other types of Leukemia, it is not likely to turn into another type of cancer. However, because CML is a cancer of the blood, it is possible for it to spread to other parts of the body, such as the liver or lungs. If this happens, it is called metastatic CML. Metastatic CML is more difficult to treat than CML that is confined to the bone marrow. While CML can be a serious disease, it is important to remember that most people with CML can be treated successfully. With early diagnosis and appropriate treatment, many people with CML can lead long and healthy lives.

What to expect when you have CML?

Chronic myeloid leukaemia (CML) is a blood cancer that usually progresses slowly. In most people with CML, the first symptom is usually an increase in the number of white blood cells. This can cause a feeling of fullness below the ribs, fatigue, and weight loss. As the disease progresses, people with CML may also experience shortness of breath, bruising or bleeding easily, and bone pain. Although CML can be a devastating diagnosis, it is important to remember that it is a treatable disease. With early diagnosis and treatment, most people with CML can expect to live long and healthy lives. The first step in managing CML is to see a doctor as soon as possible after experiencing any of the above symptoms. Once CML is diagnosed, treatment will be started immediately. The goal of treatment is to control the disease and allow people with CML to live long and healthy lives. There are a number of different treatment options available for CML, and the best treatment for each person will be determined by their individual situation. The most common treatment for CML is tyrosine kinase inhibitor (TKI) therapy. TKIs are a type of targeted therapy that work by blocking the activity of the abnormal protein that causes CML. TKI therapy is usually taken as a pill, and is often very effective at controlling the disease. Other treatment options for CML include bone marrow transplantation and stem cell transplantation. These procedures are usually only recommended for people with very advanced disease who have not responding to TKI therapy. No matter what treatment option is chosen, it is important to remember that CML is a treatable disease. With early diagnosis and treatment, most people with CML can expect to live long and healthy lives.

Are you born with CML?

There are many different types of leukaemia, but chronic myeloid leukaemia (CML) is one of the most common. So, are you born with CML? The answer is, unfortunately, we don't really know. CML is a cancer of the blood cells, and the cause is still not fully understood. However, we do know that it's not contagious, so you can't "catch" it from someone else. There are some risk factors that can make someone more likely to develop CML, such as exposure to certain chemicals or radiation, but it's not clear if these factors are the cause of the cancer or if they just make it more likely to develop. In most cases, CML seems to occur randomly, with no clear cause. This can make it difficult to prevent, and there is currently no cure. However, treatment has come a long way in recent years, and many people with CML can now manage the disease and enjoy a good quality of life.

Does CML reduce life expectancy?

CML, or chronic myeloid leukaemia, is a type of cancer that affects the blood and bones. It is a relatively rare cancer, with around 3,000 people diagnosed with it each year in the UK. CML is most common in people over the age of 60, and the average age at diagnosis is 68. CML is a slow-growing cancer, which means that it can take many years to develop and symptoms may not appear for a long time. The average life expectancy for people with

CML is around 10 years. However, this is only an average, and some people with CML can live for much longer, while others may die sooner. CML is treated with medication, and most people with CML will take medication for the rest of their life. The medication helps to control the cancer and can slow down its progression. In some cases, the medication may even cure the cancer. Although CML is a serious cancer, it is often possible to live a long and full life with the condition. With treatment, many people with CML can expect to live for many years.

Does CML have a good prognosis?

Chronic myeloid leukaemia (CML) is a type of leukaemia that gets worse slowly. It is caused by a problem with the white blood cells. CML is also called chronic myelogenous leukaemia. CML is a cancer of the blood. The word 'chronic' in chronic myeloid leukaemia means that it gets worse slowly. The word 'myeloid' refers to the cells in the bone marrow that produce blood cells. The word 'leukaemia' means cancer of the blood. CML is a type of cancer that starts in the bone marrow. The bone marrow is the soft tissue inside the bones where blood cells are made. In CML, there is a problem with the white blood cells. The white blood cells are the cells that fight infection. CML is a chronic disease, which means that it gets worse slowly. It usually takes many years for CML to get to the point where it needs to be treated. CML is a cancer that can be treated. The treatment for CML has evolved over the years, and it is now possible for most people with CML to live for many years with the disease. CML is a cancer that is diagnosed using blood tests and bone marrow tests. The treatment for CML is usually with drugs that kill the cancer cells. These drugs are called chemotherapy drugs. CML can be a serious disease, but it is important to remember that it is a treatable cancer. The prognosis for CML has improved dramatically over the past few decades, and it is now possible for most people with CML to live for many years with the disease.

Can stress cause CML?

Most people with chronic myeloid leukaemia (CML) are diagnosed in their 50s or 60s, but the condition can affect people of any age. CML is a type of blood cancer that starts in the bone marrow, where blood cells are made. In CML, a change (mutation) in a gene causes the bone marrow to produce too many white blood cells. These abnormal cells crowd out the healthy blood cells, so the blood can't do its job properly. CML is usually a slow-growing cancer. It may take months or years for symptoms to appear. In some cases, the cancer can grow quickly. The cause of CML is unknown. However, it is not caused by stress.

Does CML go to brain?

Leukaemia is a cancer of the blood cells. It is a very serious illness which can be fatal. There are two main types of leukaemia, acute and chronic. Acute leukaemia is a very serious illness which comes on very quickly. Chronic leukaemia is a less serious form of the disease which develops slowly over time. CML (chronic myeloid leukaemia) is a type of chronic leukaemia. It is a cancer of the blood cells which starts in the bone marrow. The bone marrow is the soft tissue inside the bones where blood cells are made. CML can sometimes spread to other parts of the body, such as the liver, spleen or lymph nodes. It can also sometimes spread to the brain. Thecept that CML might spread to the brain is a cause for concern for many people. However, it is important to remember that CML is a very treatable form of cancer. There are many different treatments available which are usually very effective. Most people with CML will not experience any symptoms. However, some people may experience fatigue, weight loss, night sweats or a fever. If you experience any of these symptoms, it is important to see your doctor as soon as possible. If CML is diagnosed early, it is usually very treatable.

The most common treatment for CML is medication. There are a number of different medication options available, and the right medication will be selected for each individual case. In some cases, a stem cell transplant may be recommended. This is a more aggressive treatment option which can be very effective. The prognosis for CML is generally very good. With treatment, most people with CML will live for many years. In some cases, CML can even be cured.

Though leukaemia can be difficult to treat, there are many options available and with continued research, the outlook is promising. Early detection is key, so be sure to see your doctor regularly and get any suspicious symptoms checked out right away.

Is CML the same as Leukemia?

Leukemia is a type of cancer that starts in the blood-forming cells of the bone marrow. Chronic myeloid Leukemia (CML) is a type of Leukemia that is caused by a mutation in a gene called the Philadelphia chromosome. This mutation leads to the overproduction of a protein called tyrosine-kinase. Tyrosine-kinase is a enzymes that is involved in the regulation of cell growth. The overproduction of this protein results in the excessive growth of white blood cells. White blood cells are the cells that fight infection. Although the overproduction of white blood cells helps to fight infection, it also leads to the crowding out of other blood cells, which can cause a variety of problems. CML is a slowly progressing form of Leukemia. In the early stages of CML, patients may not have any symptoms. As the disease progresses, patients may experience fatigue, weight loss, and bone pain. In the advanced stages of CML, patients may experience bleeding and bruising due to the low levels of platelets in their blood. CML is usually treated with medication, however, in some cases, patients may require a stem cell transplant. So, to answer the question, no, CML is not the same as Leukemia. CML is a type of Leukemia, but it is not the only type. There are many different types of Leukemia, each with their own set of symptoms and treatment options.

What is the survival rate for hairy cell Leukemia?

Hairy cell Leukemia (HCL) is a rare type of blood cancer that develops in the bone marrow. The average survival rate for HCL is 9 to 10 years. However, with early diagnosis and treatment, the survival rate can be as high as 20 to 30 years. The prognosis for HCL is generally good, but it can vary depending on the individual case. There are two types of HCL, classic and variant. Classic HCL is the more common type, and it tends to be more indolent (slow-growing). Variant HCL is more aggressive and has a higher rate of recurrence. The main treatment for HCL is chemotherapy. Some people may also receive radiation therapy, biologic therapy, or a stem cell transplant. The specific treatment plan will depend on the individual case. HCL is a rare cancer, and there is still much that is unknown about the disease. However, the prognosis is generally good with treatment. With early diagnosis and treatment, the survival rate for HCL can be as high as 20 to 30 years.

How serious is hairy cell Leukemia?

Leukemia is a type of cancer that starts in the blood-forming cells of the bone marrow. There are four main types of Leukemia, each of which has different characteristics. The four main types of Leukemia are: -Acute lymphocytic Leukemia (ALL) -Acute myeloid Leukemia (AML) -Chronic lymphocytic Leukemia (CLL) -Chronic myeloid Leukemia (CML) Leukemia is a cancer of the blood cells. The four main types of blood cells are: -Red blood cells -White blood cells -Platelets -Granulocytes White blood cells are further divided into two types: -Lymphocytes -Myelocytes

Lymphocytes are further divided into two types: -B lymphocytes -T lymphocytes Leukemia can be either acute or chronic. Acute Leukemia is a fast-growing cancer that occurs when there is a problem with the development of blood cells in the bone marrow. Acute Leukemia needs to be treated quickly, as it can be fatal. Chronic Leukemia is a slow-growing cancer that occurs when there is a problem with the development of blood cells in the bone marrow. Chronic Leukemia can be treated, but it is not curable. There are four main types of Leukemia, each of which has different characteristics. -Acute lymphocytic Leukemia (ALL) is the most common type of Leukemia in children. It is also the most treatable type of Leukemia. -Acute myeloid Leukemia (AML) is the most common type of Leukemia in adults. It is also the most aggressive type of Leukemia. -Chronic lymphocytic Leukemia (CLL) is the most common type of Leukemia in adults. It is a slow-growing cancer that is usually not fatal. -Chronic myeloid Leukemia (CML) is a rare type of Leukemia that is most common in adults. It is a slow-growing cancer that is usually not fatal. Leukemia is a serious disease, but it is treatable. With treatment, many people with Leukemia can expect to lead a normal life.

What is a common finding in patients with hairy cell Leukemia?

A common finding in patients with hairy cell Leukemia is a high white blood cell count. White blood cells are responsible for fighting infection, and a high count can be a sign that the body is trying to fight off an infection. Other common findings in patients with hairy cell Leukemia include fatigue, weight loss, and night sweats.

How treatable is hairy cell Leukemia?

Hairy cell Leukemia is a type of cancer that starts in the cells of the immune system. The Immune system helps to protect the body from infection and disease. The Leukemia cells grow out of control and crowd out the healthy cells in the bone marrow. The Leukemia cells may also spread to other parts of the body, such as the lymph nodes, liver, and spleen. Treatment for hairy cell Leukemia may include chemotherapy, radiation therapy, or a stem cell transplant. In some cases, the Leukemia may go into remission on its own. remission is when the cancer disappears for a period of time. The prognosis for hairy cell Leukemia is generally good. The 5-year survival rate is about 95%. This means that 95% of people with this type of Leukemia are still alive 5 years after they are diagnosed.

Why do you get hairy cell Leukemia?

Hairy cell Leukemia is a cancer of the blood and bone marrow. The cause of this type of Leukemia is not known. However, there are several risk factors that may increase your chance of developing hairy cell Leukemia. These include: • Having a family history of the disease • Being exposed to certain chemicals or radiation • Having certain medical conditions, such as autoimmune disorders • Being over the age of 60 While the exact cause of hairy cell Leukemia is not known, there are several factors that may contribute to its development. Treatment for hairy cell Leukemia often includes chemotherapy and/or radiation therapy. In some cases, a stem cell transplant may also be necessary.

Should hairy cell Leukemia patients get Covid vaccine?

Patients with hairy cell Leukemia (HCL) are at increased risk for infections due to their impaired immune systems. Because of this, HCL patients should receive the Covid vaccine when it becomes available to them. There are two types of Covid vaccines currently available: the Pfizer vaccine and the Moderna vaccine. Both of these vaccines are highly effective at preventing Covid infections. The Pfizer vaccine is 95% effective at preventing Covid infections, while the Moderna vaccine is 94% effective. There are a few potential side effects of the Covid vaccines, but they are generally mild and go away on their own. The most common side effects are pain and redness at the injection site, fatigue, headache, and muscle pain. HCL patients should talk to their doctor about whether or not they should receive the Covid vaccine. Patients who are receiving treatment for HCL may want to wait to get the vaccine until their treatment is completed. However, patients who are not currently receiving treatment may want to get the vaccine sooner. The decision of whether or not to get the Covid vaccine is a personal one. HCL patients should talk to their doctor about the risks and benefits of the vaccine before making a decision.

Leukaemia is a serious and life-threatening illness that needs urgent medical treatment. There is no one specific cause of leukaemia, but it can develop from a combination of genetic and lifestyle factors. With early diagnosis and treatment, many people with leukaemia can go on to lead long and healthy lives.

What are some fun facts about hairy cell Leukemia?

There are many different types of Leukemia, with hairy cell Leukemia (HCL) being one of the most rare. This type of cancer usually affects adults over the age of 50 and is more common in men than women. Despite its name, HCL does not cause excessive hair growth. In fact, one of the main symptoms of this type of Leukemia is weight loss and fatigue. HCL is a slow-growing cancer that is usually treatable with medication. However, in some cases, patients may need to undergo a bone marrow transplant. Here are some fun facts about this rare type of Leukemia: 1. HCL is usually diagnosed after a person presents with fatigue or weight loss. 2. This type of

Leukemia is more common in men than women. 3. HCL is a slow-growing cancer that is usually treatable with medication. 4. In some cases, patients may need to undergo a bone marrow transplant. 5. HCL is a rare type of Leukemia that affects adults over the age of 50.

What is another name for hairy cell Leukemia?

A form of Leukemia characterized by the infiltration of the bone marrow and blood with abnormal B lymphocytes. These cells have large, round nuclei with a small amount of blue-purple cytoplasm. They often have long, fingerlike processes (cytoplasmic extensions) that give them a "hairy" appearance when viewed under a microscope.

How long is chemo for hairy cell Leukemia?

There is no one answer to the question of how long chemo for hairy cell Leukemia will last, as the length of treatment will vary from person to person. Chemotherapy is often given in cycles, with each cycle consisting of a period of treatment followed by a period of rest. The length of each cycle will depend on the drugs used and how well the patient responds to treatment. Some people may only require a few cycles of chemotherapy, while others may need several months of treatment. Ultimately, the goal of chemotherapy is to kill all of the cancer cells, and the length of treatment will be determined by the efficacy of the drugs used.

How can you prevent hairy cell Leukemia?

Hairy cell Leukemia is a type of cancer that begins in the white blood cells. The cancerous cells have a hairy appearance when viewed under a microscope. There is no sure way to prevent hairy cell Leukemia. However, there are some things you can do to lower your risk. The best way to lower your risk is to avoid known risk factors. Factors that may increase your risk of hairy cell Leukemia include: * Previous treatment with certain drugs or chemicals, such as alkylating agents or topoisomerase inhibitors * Exposure to certain viruses, such as the human T-lymphotropic virus (HTLV-1) * A family history of hairy cell Leukemia There are also some things you can do to promote your overall health. A healthy lifestyle includes: * Eating a healthy diet * Getting regular exercise * Avoiding tobacco products * Managing stress * Getting enough sleep If you have any concerns about your risk of hairy cell Leukemia, talk to your doctor. They can help you make lifestyle choices that may lower your risk.

Is the COVID vaccine safe for Leukemia patients?

There is currently no evidence that Leukemia patients are at increased risk for complications from COVID-19 or that the COVID-19 vaccine is unsafe for this population. In fact, all adults, including those with Leukemia, are advised to get the COVID-19 vaccine as soon as it is available to them. While the COVID-19 pandemic has been challenging for everyone, it has been especially difficult for those with Leukemia and other chronic health conditions. People with Leukemia are at increased risk for severe illness from COVID-19, and many have had to cancel or postpone treatment due to the pandemic. The COVID-19 vaccine is an important tool to help protect people with Leukemia and other chronic health conditions from the virus. Getting the vaccine can help people with Leukemia stay healthy and reduce their risk for serious complications from COVID-19.

Does COVID vaccine affect chemotherapy?

While the full extent of the coronavirus pandemic is still unclear, scientists are already beginning to wonder how the virus will affect cancer patients. One of the most common forms of cancer, Leukemia, is treated with chemotherapy. This treatment involves using drugs to kill cancer cells. However, there is some evidence that the coronavirus may affect the efficacy of chemotherapy. A study published in the journal Nature Medicine found that the virus could reduce the number of white blood cells, which are essential for fighting infection. This could make it more difficult for cancer patients to recover from chemotherapy. There is still much unknown about the coronavirus and its effects on cancer patients. However, it is important to remain vigilant and continue to follow the advice of medical professionals.

Can Covid affect your blood count?

Covid-19 is a novel coronavirus that was first discovered in 2019. Since then, it has caused a global pandemic, with millions of people around the world infected. One of the key symptoms of Covid-19 is an abnormally high white blood cell count. White blood cells are an important part of the immune system, and help to fight off infections. In people with Covid-19, the immune system is overactive and produces too many white blood cells. This can lead to a condition called leukaemia. Leukaemia is a type of cancer that affects the blood and bone marrow. It is a very serious condition, and can be fatal if not treated early. There is currently no cure for leukaemia, but treatment can help to improve the prognosis. Covid-19 is still a relatively new virus, and more research is needed to understand the full extent of its effects on the human body. However, it is clear that it can cause serious and potentially fatal illnesses, such as leukaemia. If you think you may have Covid-19, it is important to seek medical help straight away. Early diagnosis and treatment is vital for the best chance of recovery.

In conclusion, leukaemia is a very serious illness that can have a huge impact on a person's life. It is important to be aware of the symptoms and to seek medical help as soon as possible if you think you may have the condition. With treatment, many people with leukaemia can live long and healthy lives.

Does hair fully grow back after chemo?

After chemo, hair generally starts to grow back within a few months, although it may be a different color or texture than before. It can take up to a year for hair to return to its pre-chemo state. Hair loss is one of the most common and distressing side-effects of chemotherapy. It can cause a great deal of anxiety for patients and their loved ones. Many people worry that their hair will never grow back after chemo. However, in most cases, it will. The hair loss experienced during chemo is typically temporary. In most cases, hair starts to grow back within a few months of completing treatment. It is possible for the hair to grow back a different color or texture than it was before. It may also be thinner than it was previously. It can take up to a year for hair to return to its pre-chemo state. In some cases, the hair may never quite return to its original appearance. However, it is important to remember that hair loss is only a temporary side-effect of chemo. The vast majority of people who undergo chemotherapy will eventually see their hair grow back.

Does body hair grow back after chemo?

Most people undergoing chemotherapy treatment lose all of their body hair. This includes the hair on their head, face, underarms, and pubic area. Some people also lose the hair on their legs, arms, and chest. Body hair usually starts to grow back within a few weeks after chemo has ended. The new hair may be thinner and softer than your hair was before treatment. It may also be a different color. Some people find that their new hair is curlier than it was before. It can take several months for your hair to return to its pre-treatment thickness. In the meantime, you may want to experiment with different hairstyles and products to find what works best for you. If you're not happy with the way your hair looks after chemo, talk to your doctor or healthcare team. They may be able to suggest treatments that can help.

Does body hair always grow back after chemo?

Most people undergoing chemotherapy will lose some or all of their body hair. However, it is important to remember that everyone is different and will experience different side effects. Some people may find that their body hair does not grow back after chemotherapy, while others may find that it does. It is important to talk to your doctor about the possible side effects of chemotherapy, so that you can be prepared for what to expect. If you are concerned about losing your body hair, there are a few options available to you. You may want to consider wearing a wig or headscarf, or you may choose to shave your head before starting treatment. Losing body hair can be a difficult side effect of chemotherapy, but it is important to remember that it is only temporary. Your hair will likely grow back once treatment is completed. In the meantime, there are a few options available to you to help you cope with this side effect.

What happens if you get COVID during chemo?

If you are undergoing chemotherapy for leukaemia and you contract COVID-19, it is important to seek medical advice as soon as possible. There is a risk that the virus could cause serious problems such as pneumonia, and it is also possible that the virus could interfere with your treatment. If you have any symptoms of COVID-19, such as a new continuous cough or a high temperature, you should contact your hospital immediately. You may be advised to self-isolate and to stop attending your chemotherapy appointments until you have recovered from the virus. It is important to remember that chemotherapy can weaken your immune system, making it more difficult for your body to fight off infection. This means that you are more likely to develop serious complications if you do catch COVID-19. If you are diagnosed with COVID-19, you will likely be treated with antiviral medication. You may also be given oxygen therapy if you are struggling to breathe. In severe cases, you may need to be hospitalised. It is also important to keep in mind that your cancer treatment may be delayed if you develop COVID-19. This is because it is important to rest and recover from the virus before starting treatment again. If you are worried about contracting COVID-19, there are some things you can do to reduce your risk. First, you should make sure you wash your hands regularly and avoid touching your face. You should also avoid close contact with people who are sick. Finally, you should clean and disinfect surfaces in your home.

Can Leukemia be cured?

Leukemia is a cancer of the blood cells. The main types of Leukemia are acute lymphoblastic Leukemia (ALL) and acute myeloid Leukemia (AML). Leukemia can be cured if it is found early and treated with aggressive chemotherapy. The cure rate for Leukemia has increased dramatically over the past few decades. The survival rate for children with Leukemia is now over 90%. For adults, the survival rate depends on the type of Leukemia and how early it is caught. With recent advances in treatment, the survival rate for adults with Leukemia is now 70%.

Should you vaccinate a FeLV positive cat?

There is much controversy surrounding the vaccination of felv positive cats. Some people believe that it is unnecessary and will only make the cat sicker, while others believe that it is important to protect the cat from other diseases. So, what is the right answer? The feline Leukemia virus (FeLV) is a serious and often fatal disease in cats. It is most commonly spread through close contact with other cats, so cats who live in close quarters with other cats (such as in a shelter or rescue) are at especially high risk. There is no cure for FeLV, so once a cat becomes infected, the virus will remain in their system for their entire life. There are two types of vaccines available for FeLV: an initial vaccine and a booster vaccine. The initial vaccine is given in two doses, given two to four weeks apart. After the initial vaccines, cats should receive a booster vaccine every year. Cats who are infected with FeLV can spread the virus to other cats through close contact, such as sharing food, water, litter boxes, or beds. The virus can also be spread through blood transfusions, contaminated needles, or mother-to-kitten transfer during pregnancy or delivery. There are several things to consider before deciding whether or not to vaccinate a FeLV positive cat. The first is the cat's age. Kittens are much more likely to develop serious health problems from the virus than adults, so it is generally recommended that all kittens be vaccinated. Another factor to consider is the cat's lifestyle. Cats who live indoors or who have limited contact with other cats are at a lower risk of contracting FeLV than cats who go outdoors or who have a lot of contact with other cats. Finally, you should talk to your veterinarian about the risks and benefits of vaccinating a FeLV positive cat. They will be able to help you make the best decision for your cat's individual situation.

Can I have flu jab while on chemo?

Can I have flu jab while on chemo? If you are undergoing chemotherapy, you may be wondering if you can still get the flu jab. The good news is that you can! In general, it is recommended that everyone six months of age and older get the flu jab, especially those with certain medical conditions like cancer. Even though chemotherapy can weaken your immune system, the flu jab is still safe and effective for people undergoing treatment. In fact, it is especially important for people with cancer to get the flu jab since they are at an increased risk of developing complications from the flu. If you are unsure whether or not you should get the flu jab, speak to your doctor or cancer care team. They will be able to advise you on whether or not the flu jab is right for you.

Leukaemia is a serious disease that can be fatal. However, with early diagnosis and treatment, many people with leukaemia can lead long and healthy lives.

Can COVID vaccine lower red blood cell count?

COVID-19 has been a global pandemic for over a year now. The virus has claimed the lives of over 2.5 million people worldwide. With the global community desperate for a solution, scientists have been working around the clock to develop a vaccine. The first vaccine was approved for use in December 2020 and since then, over 100 million doses have been administered. There is now some evidence to suggest that the vaccine may have an unintended side effect - it may lower red blood cell count. A study published in the New England Journal of Medicine found that a small number of people who had received the vaccine developed a condition called vaccine-induced immune thrombotic thrombocytopenia (VITT). This condition can lead to a decrease in red blood cells, which can in turn lead to fatigue, shortness of breath and an increased risk of infection. While the risk of developing VITT is low (estimated at around 1 in a million), it is important to be aware of the potential side effects of the vaccine. If you experience any of the above symptoms after receiving the vaccine, you should contact your doctor immediately.

What are examples of myelodysplastic syndromes?

Myelodysplastic syndromes (MDS) are a group of blood disorders that affect the bone marrow and blood. In MDS, the bone marrow does not make enough healthy blood cells. MDS can develop into acute myeloid Leukemia (AML). There are many different types of MDS. The most common type is refractory anemia (RA). RA is a condition in which the bone marrow does not make enough red blood cells. People with RA may have fatigue, shortness of breath, and pale skin. Other types of MDS include: -Refractory anemia with ringed sideroblasts (RARS) -Refractory anemia with excess blasts (RAEB) -Refractory anemia with excess blasts in transformation (RAEB-T) -Chronic myelomonocytic Leukemia (CMML) -Myelodysplastic syndrome associated with a previous chemotherapy treatment (MDS-CT) Treatment for MDS often depends on the type of MDS. People with RA may not need treatment. People with RARS, RAEB, or RAEB-T may need blood transfusions or treatment with drugs that stimulate the production of blood cells. People with CMML may need treatment with drugs that kill cancer cells. People with MDS-CT often need the same treatment that they received for their original cancer.

How serious is myelodysplastic syndrome?

MDS is a cancer of the blood and bone marrow. It is a rare disease that affects mostly older adults. The cause of MDS is unknown. MDS is a serious disease. It can be hard to treat, and it can be fatal. The disease can progress quickly, or it can take many years to develop. There are different types of MDS. Some types are more serious than others. The type of MDS you have, your age, and your overall health will affect how serious your disease is. MDS can be hard to diagnose. The symptoms can be subtle, and they can vary from person to person. Often, MDS is diagnosed after a blood test shows abnormal blood cells. If you have MDS, you will need treatment. The type of treatment you need will depend on the type of

MDS you have, how serious your disease is, and your age and overall health. Treatment can include blood transfusions, chemotherapy, and stem cell transplants. MDS is a serious disease. It can be hard to treat, and it can be fatal. If you have MDS, you will need treatment. The type of treatment you need will depend on the type of MDS you have, how serious your disease is, and your age and overall health.

What causes myelodysplastic syndrome?

There are many different possible causes of myelodysplastic syndrome (MDS), and doctors often cannot identify a specific cause. However, there are some known risk factors that may play a role in the development of MDS. One possible cause of MDS is exposure to certain chemicals or radiation. Chemicals that are known to be risky include certain chemotherapy drugs used to treat cancer, and those used in the production of vinyl chloride (used in the manufacturing of PVC plastic). Ionising radiation, such as that used for cancer treatment, can also damage the cells that produce blood. Another potential cause of MDS is having a blood relative with the condition. This suggests that there may be a genetic component to the development of MDS. In fact, studies have found that people with certain genetic mutations are more likely to develop MDS. These mutations affect proteins involved in the regulation of cell division, and may cause the cells to divide abnormally. Other possible risk factors for MDS include being elderly, having certain blood disorders, and having had a bone marrow transplant. However, it is important to remember that many people with these risk factors will not go on to develop MDS. Overall, the exact cause of MDS is often unknown. However, there are some known risk factors that may play a role in its development.

Is myelodysplasia a form of Leukemia?

Myelodysplastic syndromes (MDS) are a heterogeneous group of myeloid neoplasms characterized by ineffective hematopoiesis and variable degrees of cell differentiation. MDS can progress to acute myeloid Leukemia (AML), and thus these two groups of disorders are considered together in this section. The World Health Organization (WHO) classifies MDS and AML according to morphologic, immunophenotypic, cytogenetic, and molecular features. MDS are clonal hematopoietic stem cell disorders characterized by ineffective hematopoiesis, bone marrow failure, and peripheral cytopenias. The cytopenias are the result of impaired production of one or more hematopoietic lineages. The morphologic features of MDS are variable, and range from being barely noticeable to very prominent. The most common feature is dyserythropoiesis, which can range from mild to severe. Other features include ringed sideroblasts, endogenous erythroid colonies, myeloid hyperplasia, and dysmegakaryopoiesis. In general, the greater the degree of cytopenias, the more likely it is that the morphologic features will be prominent. MDS can be further classified according to the presence or absence of blasts in the bone marrow. If blasts make up 5% or more of the cells in the bone marrow, the disorder is classified as AML. If the blasts make up less than 5% of the cells in the bone marrow, the disorder is classified as MDS. The vast majority of MDS cases are diagnosed when the blasts make up less than 5% of the cells in the bone marrow. The cause of MDS is unknown. However, there are several risk factors that have been associated with an increased risk of developing MDS. These include exposure to certain chemicals (such as benzene), radiation therapy, and certain viral infections (such as human T-lymphotropic virus type 1). In addition, MDS is more common in people with certain genetic disorders, such as Down syndrome. There is no cure for MDS. However, treatment can help to control the symptoms and improve the quality of life. Treatment options include blood transfusions, medications (such as erythropoietin and granulocyte-colony stimulating factor), and stem cell transplantation. Is myelodysplasia a form of Leukemia? Myelodysplastic syndromes (MDS) are a heterogeneous group of myeloid neoplasms characterized by ineffective hematopoiesis and variable degrees of cell differentiation. MDS can progress to acute myeloid Leukemia (AML), and thus these two groups of disorders are considered together in this section. The World Health Organization (WHO) classifies MDS and AML according to morph

What is early stage myelodysplastic syndrome?

Myelodysplastic syndrome (MDS) is a cancer of the blood and bone marrow. It is a type of leukaemia. MDS is characterised by the production of abnormal blood cells. These abnormal blood cells do not function properly and do not mature. MDS can progress to acute myeloid leukaemia (AML). MDS is a cancer of the blood and bone marrow. The bone marrow is the spongy tissue inside the bones where blood cells are made. MDS is a type of leukaemia. Leukaemia is a cancer of the blood cells. MDS is characterised by the production of abnormal blood cells. These abnormal blood cells do not function properly and do not mature. MDS can progress to acute myeloid leukaemia (AML). MDS is a slowly progressing cancer. In the early stages, MDS may not cause any symptoms. As the disease progresses, symptoms may develop. These can include: fatigue, breathlessness, Pallor (paleness), increased risk of infection, bleeding, and anaemia. If you experience any of these symptoms, please see your doctor. MDS is diagnosed through a combination of medical history, physical examination, blood tests, bone marrow biopsy, and cytogenetic testing. A bone marrow biopsy is a procedure where a sample of bone marrow is taken from the hip bone. This sample is then analysed in a laboratory. Cytogenetic testing is a type of genetic testing. This test looks for changes in the chromosomes of the blood cells. There is no one specific cause of MDS. However, there are some risk factors that may increase your chance of developing MDS. These include: exposure to certain chemicals, such as benzene; radiation therapy;

certain medications, such as chemotherapy; smoking; and family history. There is no cure for MDS. However, treatment can help to control the disease and ease symptoms. Treatment options include: blood transfusions, iron chelation therapy, stem cell transplant, and medication. Blood transfusions can help to relieve symptoms of anaemia. Iron chelation therapy is a treatment that removes excess iron from the body. This can be helpful for people with MDS who have had multiple blood transfusions. A stem cell transplant is a procedure where stem cells are transplanted from a donor into the patient. This can be a cure for MDS, but it is a risky procedure. Medication can be used to control symptoms and slow the progression of the disease. MDS is a cancer of the blood and bone marrow. It is a type of leukaemia. MDS is characterised by the production of abnormal blood cells. These abnormal blood cells do not function properly and do not mature. MDS can progress to acute myeloid leukaemia (AML). MDS is a slowly progressing cancer. In the early stages, MDS may

Can you live a full life with MDS?

The answer to this question is not straightforward, as it largely depends on the individual case. MDS is a cancer of the blood cells, which can progress quickly or slowly, and affect different people in different ways. In some cases, people with MDS will require treatment (usually with chemotherapy) which can be successful in controlling the disease and enabling people to live full and active lives. In other cases, the disease may progress more quickly and cause more serious problems such as respiratory failure or organ damage, which can shorten life expectancy. However, it is important to remember that MDS is a complex and variable disease, and so it is not possible to make definitive statements about life expectancy or quality of life for all patients. Some people with MDS live for many years with the disease, while others may die from it within a few months. It is therefore important to discuss prognosis and treatment options with a specialist doctor who can tailor recommendations to the individual patient.

Leukaemia is a type of cancer that affects the blood and bone marrow. It is a complex and serious disease that requires expert care and treatment. The outlook for people with leukaemia varies depending on the individual situation. With advances in treatment and early diagnosis, the prognosis for people with leukaemia is improving.

What are signs that MDS is progressing?

There are a few different things that can happen when MDS progresses. The first is that your anemia may worsen. This means that you may have more fatigue and need more blood transfusions than you did before. You may also notice that you are bruising or bleeding more easily. Another sign that MDS is progressing is that your white blood cell count may go up. This can lead to infections, which can be serious. You may also have more mouth sores. Finally, your platelet count may go down. This can cause easy bruising, bleeding, and fatigue. If you notice any of these changes, it is important to tell your doctor right away. They will be able to help you manage your condition and make sure that you are as comfortable as possible.

Is myelodysplastic syndrome always fatal?

MDS is a cancer of the blood and bone marrow. The bone marrow is the spongy tissue inside some of your bones where blood cells are made. MDS is a type of cancer that affects the production of blood cells in the bone marrow. MDS is a type of cancer that can be fatal. MDS is a cancer of the blood and bone marrow. The bone marrow is the spongy tissue inside some of your bones where blood cells are made. MDS is a type of cancer that affects the production of blood cells in the bone marrow. MDS is often diagnosed when a person has a low number of red blood cells, white blood cells, or platelets in their blood. A diagnosis of MDS can also be made if abnormal blood cells are found in the bone marrow. MDS is a type of cancer that can be fatal. There are different types of MDS, and the type you have affects your outlook. Some types of MDS can be treated and cured. Other types are more difficult to treat and can be fatal. If you have MDS, it is important to talk to your doctor about your treatment options. Some types of MDS can be treated with chemotherapy or bone marrow transplants. These treatments can be effective, but they are not always successful. MDS is a type of cancer that can be fatal. Although MDS can be a serious illness, many people with MDS live long and healthy lives. The outlook for someone with MDS depends on the type of MDS they have. Some types of MDS are more difficult to treat than others. MDS is a type of cancer that can be fatal.

What is the most common finding in myelodysplastic syndrome?

There are a few key findings that are generally seen in myelodysplastic syndrome (MDS), but the most common finding is typically anaemia. This is often due to a decrease in red blood cells, and can cause fatigue, breathlessness, and an increased heart rate. There may also be a decrease in white blood cells, which can lead to an increased risk of infection. Platelet levels may also be decreased, which can cause easy bruising or bleeding. In some cases, there may also be an increase in blasts (immature blood cells) in the bone marrow.

Does myelodysplasia run in families?

A diagnosis of myelodysplasia (MDS) can be devastating for patients and their families. The potential for the disease to progress to Leukemia is a major concern. Many people with MDS have questions about the risk of the disease being passed on to their children. There is currently no known way to prevent MDS from developing. However, the risk of developing MDS appears to be lower in people who have family members with the disease. This may be due to genetic factors. There is no clear evidence that MDS is passed down from generation to generation in families. However, some studies have shown that people with a family history of MDS are more likely to develop the disease themselves. This suggests that there may be a genetic link. MDS is a complex disease and the exact cause is unknown. However, it is clear that genetics plays a role. If you have a family member with MDS, you may be at increased risk of developing the disease yourself.

Does MDS start suddenly?

MDS is a blood cancer that can progress quickly or slowly. In some cases, MDS can transform into acute leukaemia, which progresses quickly and is more difficult to treat. The speed at which MDS progresses varies from person to person. MDS can start suddenly, or it can develop over time. There is not always one clear answer when it comes to the question of whether or not MDS starts suddenly. In some instances, people with MDS may notice a rapid decrease in their energy levels or an increase in their bruising or bleeding. Others may not experience any symptoms at all until their MDS is detected during a routine blood test. Even though MDS can technically start suddenly, it is more often the case that MDS progresses slowly over time. This is why it is important for people with MDS to see their doctor regularly and have any new or unusual symptoms checked out. By catching MDS early, treatment can be started sooner and may be more effective.

What causes death in MDS patients?

Although myelodysplastic syndromes (MDS) are a heterogeneous group of disorders, they all share a common myeloid cell marrow dysfunction that predisposes patients to acquiring certain infections, bleeding problems, and anemia. In terms of death rates, patients with MDS have a higher risk of mortality than the general population. The 5-year overall survival rate for patients diagnosed with MDS is approximately 27%. This is in contrast to the general population, where the 5-year overall survival rate is approximately 60%. There are several potential causes of death in patients with MDS. One of the most common is infection. This is because patients with MDS often have a weakened immune system, which makes them more susceptible to contracting infections. Infections can range from minor, such as a cold, to more serious, such as pneumonia. Another potential cause of death in patients with MDS is bleeding. This is because patients with MDS often have low platelet counts, which can lead to bleeding. Bleeding can range from minor, such as a nosebleed, to more serious, such as internal bleeding. Anemia is another potential cause of death in patients with MDS. This is because patients with MDS often have low red blood cell counts, which can lead to anemia. Anemia can range from mild, where patients may experience fatigue, to more severe, where patients may need a blood transfusion. Lastly, patients with MDS may die from complications related to their disorder. For example, patients with MDS may develop certain cancers, such as acute myeloid Leukemia (AML), as a result of their disorder. Patients with MDS may also develop other complications, such as heart failure, as a result of their disorder.

How is MDS treated in the elderly?

MDS is a type of cancer that affects the blood and bone marrow. The most common type of MDS is acute myeloid Leukemia (AML), which is a cancer of the white blood cells. MDS can also be a form of chronic lymphocytic Leukemia (CLL), which is a cancer of the lymphocytes. MDS is more common in adults over the age of 60. There are many different ways to treat MDS, and the treatment depends on the type of MDS, the stage of the disease, and the overall health of the patient. The most common treatment for MDS is chemotherapy. This is a treatment that uses drugs to kill cancer cells. Chemotherapy can be given in many different ways, such as intravenously (into a vein), orally (by mouth), or topically (applied to the skin). Other treatments for MDS include radiation therapy, stem cell transplant, and targeted therapy. Radiation therapy uses high-energy beams to kill cancer cells. Stem cell transplant is a treatment that replaces the stem cells in the bone marrow with healthy stem cells from a donor. Targeted therapy is a treatment that uses drugs or other substances to target and kill cancer cells. The treatment for MDS is decided by the doctor, and it is important to make sure that all options are considered. The side effects of each treatment should also be taken into account. MDS is a serious disease, and the treatment should be chosen based on what is best for the patient.

Leukaemia is a type of cancer that affects the white blood cells. It is the most common type of blood cancer in children and young adults.

What are the symptoms of myelodysplasia?

Leukaemia is a cancer of the blood cells. The four main types of leukaemia are: - Acute lymphoblastic leukaemia (ALL) - Acute myeloid leukaemia (AML) - Chronic lymphocytic leukaemia (CLL) - Chronic myeloid leukaemia (CML) Leukaemia can occur at any age, but is most common in children and older adults. The symptoms of leukaemia vary depending on the type of leukaemia. Acute lymphoblastic leukaemia (ALL) The symptoms of ALL develop quickly over a few weeks and include: - Frequent infections - Easy bruising or bleeding - Fatigue - Weakness - Shortness of breath - Loss of appetite - Weight loss - Bone and joint pain - Enlarged lymph nodes, liver or spleen Acute myeloid leukaemia (AML) The symptoms of AML develop over a few weeks or months and include: - Frequent infections - Easy bruising or bleeding - Fatigue - Weakness - Shortness of breath - Loss of appetite - Weight loss - Bone and joint pain - Enlarged liver or spleen - Swelling of the gums Chronic lymphocytic leukaemia (CLL) The symptoms of CLL develop slowly over months or years and include: - Enlarged lymph nodes - fatigue - Weakness - Weight loss - Easy bruising or bleeding - Infections Chronic myeloid leukaemia (CML) The symptoms of CML develop slowly over months or years and include: - Enlarged spleen - fatigue - Weakness -Weight loss - Easy bruising or bleeding If you have any of these symptoms, it is important to see a doctor so that they can perform some tests to rule out other conditions.

Does chemotherapy work on MDS?

MDS is a type of cancer that begins in the bone marrow. The bone marrow is the spongy tissue inside the bones where blood cells are made. MDS is a cancer of the blood-forming cells. Chemotherapy is a treatment that uses drugs to kill cancer cells. Chemotherapy does work on MDS, but the response rates are lower than for other types of cancer. In a study of people with MDS, the overall response rate to chemotherapy was 26 percent. This means that 26 out of 100 people with MDS had their cancer go into remission after treatment with chemotherapy. However, the remission rates varied depending on the type of chemotherapy used. There are many different types of chemotherapy drugs, and each type works differently. Some chemotherapy drugs work by targeting cancer cells that are dividing quickly. Other drugs work by targeting all cells that are dividing, including normal cells. The side effects of chemotherapy are caused by the damage to normal cells. The most common side effects of chemotherapy are fatigue, nausea and vomiting, problems with blood counts, and hair loss. Most of these side effects go away after treatment is over. Some side effects, such as problems with blood counts, may last longer. Some chemotherapy drugs can also cause long-term side effects, such as secondary cancers. Despite the side effects, chemotherapy is often the best treatment option for MDS. In some cases, a stem cell transplant may be an option for people with MDS. A stem cell transplant is a treatment that uses healthy blood cells from a donor to replace the blood-forming cells in the bone marrow. This treatment is often used for people with MDS who have not responded to other treatments.

What should I avoid if I have MDS?

If you have myelodysplastic syndrome (MDS), there are certain things you should avoid to help keep your condition under control. For example, you should avoid exposure to chemicals and radiation, as these can worsen your condition. You should also avoid smoking, as this can also aggravate your condition. Alcohol should also be avoided, as it can interfere with your treatment. Finally, you should also avoid stress, as this can trigger a flare-up of your symptoms.

Can MDS be cured with chemo?

MDS is a type of blood cancer that can be treated with chemotherapy. The main goal of treatment is to control the cancer and relieve symptoms. MDS can be cured with chemotherapy in some cases, but the chance of cure depends on the type of MDS and the response to treatment. Some people with MDS may need multiple courses of chemotherapy, and some may need stem cell transplant. The side effects of chemotherapy can be severe, but there are ways to manage them.

What age group gets MDS?

MDS is most common in older adults. The average age of diagnosis is 71. However, MDS can occur in people of any age. In general, the risk of MDS increases with age. MDS is a cancer of the blood and bone marrow. It is caused by a problem with the blood-forming cells in the bone marrow. The bone marrow is the spongy tissue inside bones that makes blood cells. In MDS, the blood-forming cells do not mature normally. This results in fewer, abnormal blood cells being made. MDS is a type of cancer that can be difficult to diagnose early. This is because the early symptoms are often vague and nonspecific. They can also be caused by other conditions. For example, fatigue and shortness of breath are common symptoms of MDS. But they can also be caused by other conditions that are not cancer, such as anemia or a viral infection. If you have any symptoms that concern you, it is important to see your doctor. They can perform tests to check for MDS.

Can MDS lead to other cancers?

MDS is a cancer of the blood and bone marrow. It is a type of Leukemia, which is a cancer of the blood cells. MDS can lead to other cancers, such as Leukemia, lymphoma, and myeloma.

Does MDS cause pain?

MDS is a cancer of the blood and bone marrow. The main symptom of MDS is fatigue. However, some people with MDS may also have shortness of breath, easy bruising or bleeding, fever, or weight loss. Some people with MDS may also experience pain. Pain is a common symptom of cancer, and can be caused by the cancer itself, or by treatments for the cancer. Cancer pain can be caused by pressure on the nerves or organs, inflammation, or by the cancer growing into the bones. Treatments for MDS can also cause pain. For example, chemotherapy can cause pain in the hands and feet, and radiation therapy can cause pain in the area being treated. There are several ways to manage cancer pain. The first step is to identify the cause of the pain. Once the cause is identified, the healthcare team can recommend the best treatment for the pain. Pain medication can be used to help control the pain. In some cases, other treatments, such as physical therapy, acupuncture, or electrical nerve stimulation, may be recommended. Cancer pain is different for everyone. Some people have mild pain that can be managed with over-the-counter medication. Others have more severe pain that requires stronger medication. The important thing is to talk to your healthcare team about the pain you are experiencing. They can help you find the best way to manage your pain.

As researchers continue to unlock the secrets of cancer cells, they are also discovering more and more about how to effectively treat leukaemia. While there is still no cure for leukaemia, treatments are becoming more and more effective, giving patients hope for a longer and healthier life.

What part of the body does MDS affect?

MDS, or myelodysplastic syndrome, is a type of cancer that affects the blood and bone marrow. The bone marrow is the soft tissue inside the bones where blood cells are made. MDS can cause the bone marrow to make too few blood cells, which can lead to problems such as fatigue, shortness of breath, and an increased risk of infection. MDS can also cause the bone marrow to make abnormal blood cells, which can cause problems such as bleeding and blood clots. MDS is a rare cancer that usually affects older adults. It is most common in people over the age of 60. However, MDS can occur in people of any age. The cause of MDS is not known. However, there are some risk factors that may increase your chance of developing MDS. These include: • Having certain blood disorders, such as thalassemia or myelodysplasia • Having certain genetic conditions, such as Down syndrome or Diamond-Blackfan syndrome • Being exposed to certain chemicals, such as benzene • Having certain medical conditions, such as aplastic anaemia or lupus • Having received certain cancer treatments, such as radiation therapy or chemotherapy If you have any of these risk factors, it does not mean that you will develop MDS. However, it is important to discuss your risk factors with your doctor. There is no cure for MDS. However, treatment can often help manage the symptoms and side effects of the disease. The type of treatment you receive will depend on the severity of your disease and your overall health. Treatment options for MDS include: • Blood transfusions: This can help treat anaemia by replacing missing or damaged red blood cells. • Iron chelation therapy: This can help treat anaemia by removing excess iron from the body. Iron can build up in the body if you receive frequent blood transfusions. • Stem cell transplant: This is a treatment that can cure MDS. However, it is a very risky procedure. It is usually only an option for people who are under the age of 60 and who have a donor who is a close match. MDS is a serious disease that can be life-threatening. However, with treatment, many people with MDS are able to live long and healthy lives.

What are the symptoms of myeloproliferative disorder?

There are a range of symptoms associated with myeloproliferative disorders, and these can vary depending on the specific disorder. However, some common symptoms include: - feeling tired and weak - easy bruising or bleeding - shortness of breath - feeling full after only eating a small amount - weight loss - bone pain - vision problems If you have any of these symptoms, it's important to see your doctor so they can rule out other potential causes and start appropriate treatment.

How serious is myeloproliferative disorder?

Myeloproliferative disorder is a type of cancer that affects the blood and bone marrow. It is a serious condition that can be life-threatening. The most common symptom of myeloproliferative disorder is fatigue. Other symptoms may include: • Feeling tired all the time • Shortness of breath • Easily bruisable • Excessive bleeding • Anemia • Weight loss • Bone pain If you have any of these symptoms, it is important to see your doctor as soon as possible. Myeloproliferative disorder is diagnosed through a combination of physical examination, blood tests, and bone marrow biopsy. Treatment for myeloproliferative disorder may include medication, radiation therapy, and/or stem cell transplant.

Is myeloproliferative disorders a cancer?

Myeloproliferative disorders (MPDs) are a type of cancer that affect the blood and bone marrow. The three main types of MPDs are myelofibrosis, polycythemia vera, and essential thrombocythemia. MPDs can be difficult to diagnose because they typically do not cause symptoms in the early stages. When symptoms do develop, they can be mild and mimic other conditions. MPDs develop when the body produces too many white blood cells, red blood cells, or platelets. This overproduction can cause the bone marrow to become overloaded and unable to function properly. The excess cells can also crowd out healthy blood cells and prevent them from doing their job. As the disease progresses, it can lead to anemia, bleeding, and fatigue. There is no cure for MPDs, but treatments are available to help control the disease and ease symptoms. Treatment options include medication, radiation therapy, and stem cell transplant. MPDs are rare diseases that affect less than 1% of the population. While there is no sure way to prevent these cancers, there are some risk factors that may increase your chances of developing an MPD. Risk factors include exposure to certain chemicals, radiation, or viruses. MPDs are also more common in people with certain genetic disorders, such as Down syndrome.

What is the most common myeloproliferative disorder?

Leukaemia is a cancer of the blood cells. The most common type of leukaemia is acute lymphoblastic leukaemia (ALL). ALL is a cancer of the lymphocytes, which are a type of white blood cell. Lymphocytes are made in the bone marrow and are vital for the body's immune system. They help to fight infection by producing antibodies. In ALL, the lymphocytes grow out of control and crowd out the healthy blood cells in the bone marrow. This can lead to a decrease in the production of healthy blood cells, which can make people with ALL susceptible to infection. ALL can affect people of any age, but is most common in children under the age of 5. It is also more common in boys than girls. In the UK, around 400 children are diagnosed with ALL each year. There are several subtypes of ALL, which are determined by the type of lymphocyte that is affected. The most common subtype in children is B-cell ALL. The symptoms of ALL can vary depending on the type of leukaemia and how advanced it is. Some common symptoms include: - fatigue - breathlessness - easy bruising or bleeding - bone or joint pain - fever - weight loss. If you or your child has any of these symptoms, it is important to see a doctor as soon as possible. ALL is usually diagnosed with a blood test and a bone marrow biopsy. A bone marrow biopsy is a procedure to remove a small sample of bone marrow from the hipbone. The sample is then examined under a microscope to look for Leukemia cells. Once ALL is diagnosed, treatment can start immediately. The main treatment for ALL is chemotherapy, which uses drugs to kill the Leukemia cells. Chemotherapy is usually given in cycles, with each cycle lasting for a few weeks. After finishing chemotherapy, people with ALL will usually have a bone marrow transplant. This is a procedure to replace the bone marrow with healthy bone marrow from a donor.

A bone marrow transplant can often cure ALL. In some cases, people with ALL may also need to have radiation therapy. Radiation therapy uses high-energy rays to kill Leukemia cells. The prognosis for ALL depends on many factors, such as the type of leukaemia, the age of the person and how well they respond to treatment. With treatment, the survival rate for children with ALL is now around 85%.

How long can you live with myeloproliferative disorder?

The myeloproliferative disorders are a group of related disorders where the bone marrow doesn't produce the normal mixture of blood cells. Instead, it produces too many of one type of blood cell. This can cause problems with bleeding, bruising, fatigue and an increased risk of infections. The myeloproliferative disorders include: • Chronic myeloid leukaemia (CML) • Polycythaemia vera (PV) • Essential thrombocythaemia (ET) • Myelofibrosis (MF) The myeloproliferative disorders are all treatable, but not curable. The aim of treatment is to relieve symptoms and prevent complications. With treatment, most people with a myeloproliferative disorder can expect to live for many years. The life expectancy for people with CML has increased dramatically since the introduction of targeted therapy in the early 2000s. Before targeted therapy, the average life expectancy for people with CML was 3-5 years from diagnosis. With targeted therapy, the average life expectancy is now around 20 years. People with PV have a life expectancy that is similar to the general population. However, people with PV are at an increased risk of developing blood clots. This can lead to heart attacks, strokes and pulmonary embolism. Similarly, people with ET have a life expectancy that is similar to the general population. However, people with ET are at an increased risk of developing blood clots. This can lead to heart attacks, strokes and pulmonary embolism. The life expectancy for people with MF depends on how advanced the disease is at diagnosis. People with early-stage MF have a life expectancy that is similar to the general population. However, people with late-stage MF have a life expectancy of 5-10 years. In conclusion, the myeloproliferative disorders are treatable, but not curable. The life expectancy for people with a myeloproliferative disorder depends on the specific disorder. With treatment, most people with a myeloproliferative disorder can expect to live for many years.

What is the survival rate of myeloproliferative?

MPDs are a group of disorders of the blood cells. In MPDs, the cells in the bone marrow that produce blood cells (including white blood cells, red blood cells, and platelets) grow abnormally. This results in too many blood cells being produced. The overproduction of blood cells can cause problems with the blood clotting process, as well as with the function of the immune system. MPDs can also cause problems with the organs that filter the blood, such as the liver and spleen. The survival rate for myeloproliferative disorders (MPDs) varies depending on the type of MPD. For example, the 5-year survival rate for chronic myelogenous Leukemia (CML) is approximately 80%. However, the 5-year survival rate for myelofibrosis (MF) is only approximately 10%. The overall survival rate for MPDs has improved over the last few decades due to advances in treatment. However, there is still no cure for MPDs. The goal of treatment is to control the overproduction of blood cells and to relieve symptoms. Treatment may include medication, such as chemotherapy, or a stem cell transplant.

Leukemia is a serious disease that can be fatal. Early diagnosis and treatment is essential for the best possible outcome. There is no one definitive cause of Leukemia, but it is thought to be caused by a combination of genetic and environmental factors. Treatment for Leukemia can be complex and expensive, but there are many organizations and resources available to help patients and their families cope with the disease.

What is the difference between Leukemia and myeloproliferative disorder?

Leukemia is a cancer of the blood cells, characterized by an abnormal increase in the number of white blood cells in the body. Myeloproliferative disorders are a group of blood disorders that affect the bone marrow, the tissue where blood cells are produced. Leukemia can be either acute or chronic. Acute Leukemia is a rapidly progressing form of the disease, while chronic Leukemia progresses more slowly. Myeloproliferative disorders are also classified according to their rate of progression, with chronic myeloproliferative disorders progressing more slowly than acute myeloproliferative disorders. The main difference between Leukemia and myeloproliferative disorders is the type of blood cell that is affected. Leukemia affects the white blood cells, while myeloproliferative disorders affect the red blood cells and platelets. Additionally, Leukemia is a cancer of the blood cells, while myeloproliferative disorders are not considered cancers. Leukemia is treated with chemotherapy, radiation, or a bone marrow transplant. Myeloproliferative disorders are treated with medication, and in some cases, a bone marrow transplant.

How do you test for myeloproliferative disorder?

A blood test is generally the first step in diagnosing myeloproliferative disorder (MPD). This is because MPD is a blood cancer, which means that it affects the cells in the blood. There are several different types of blood tests that can be used to diagnose MPD. The most common is a complete blood count (CBC). This test measures the number of red blood cells, white blood cells, and platelets in the blood. People with MPD usually have an abnormally high number of white blood cells. Other tests that may be used to diagnose MPD include a bone marrow biopsy and a genetic test. A bone marrow biopsy is a procedure in which a small sample of bone marrow is taken from the hip bone. This sample is then examined under a microscope to look for abnormal cells. A genetic test looks for changes in the genes that are associated with MPD. MPD is usually diagnosed by a hematologist, a doctor who specializes in blood disorders.

How common is myeloproliferative disorders?

The myeloproliferative disorders (MPDs) are a group of diseases in which the bone marrow and blood cells produce too many of one or more cell types. MPDs can be acute or chronic. They can be life-threatening, but with the right treatment, most people with MPDs can lead long and healthy lives. MPDs are not common. In the United States, they affect about 1 in 500,000 people. But because there are different types of MPDs, and because not all people with MPDs have the same symptoms, it can be hard to know how many people have these disorders. MPDs can happen to anyone, but they are more common in people who have a family history of the disorder. They are also more common in men than in women.

Is myeloproliferative disorder rare?

MPD represents a group of hematologic disorders that are characterized by the abnormal production of one or more myeloid cell lineages in the bone marrow. MPDs can be either acquired or inherited, and while they are considered rare diseases, their incidence is likely underdiagnosed and underreported. The most common MPDs are essential thrombocythemia (ET), polycythemia vera (PV), and myelofibrosis (MF). MPDs are often difficult to diagnose due to their varied and nonspecific symptoms. MPDs can present with fatigue, Easy bruising, epistaxis, gingival bleeding, headache, and dizziness secondary to anemia or thrombocytopenia. PV and ET can also cause erythromelalgia, livedo reticularis, pruritus, and digital ulcers. MF can cause splenomegaly, fatigue, anorexia, and weight loss. As MPDs progress, they can lead to leukostasis, thrombosis, and organ damage. The cause of MPDs is still largely unknown, though there are some risk factors that have been identified. MPDs can be caused by exposure to certain chemicals, such as benzene, as well as ionizing radiation. Additionally, MPDs can be caused by mutations in certain genes, such as JAK2, CALR, and MPL. Acquired MPDs are more common in the elderly, while inherited MPDs can occur at any age. There is no one-size-fits-all treatment for MPDs, as the best course of action depends on the specific disorder and how advanced it is. PV and ET can often be managed with lifestyle changes and medications to control symptoms. MF is generally more difficult to treat, and may require a bone marrow transplant. MPDs are rare diseases, but they are serious conditions that can be difficult to diagnose and treat. If you think you or someone you know may have a MPD, it is important to see a doctor for a proper evaluation.

What is the average age of myelofibrosis?

The average age of myelofibrosis is approximately 60 years old. Myelofibrosis is a rare form of cancer that affects the bone marrow and blood. The average age of myelofibrosis patients is typically older than those with other forms of Leukemia. The average age of myelofibrosis patients is also generally higher than the average age of Leukemia patients. There are a number of factors that may contribute to the higher average age of myelofibrosis patients. One factor is that myelofibrosis is often diagnosed at a later stage than other forms of Leukemia. This is due to the fact that myelofibrosis often does not present with any symptoms until the disease is quite advanced. Another factor that may contribute to the higher average age of myelofibrosis patients is that myelofibrosis is a slow-growing form of cancer. This means that patients may live for many years with the disease before it is diagnosed. Myelofibrosis is a serious form of cancer that can cause a number of health problems. It is important for patients to be aware of the symptoms of myelofibrosis and to seek medical help if they experience any of them.

What is the life expectancy of a person with myelofibrosis?

Myelofibrosis is a rare blood cancer that occurs when the bone marrow becomes scarred and doesn't produce enough healthy blood cells. This can lead to a range of symptoms, including fatigue, anaemia and bone pain. In some cases, myelofibrosis can progress to Leukemia. The life expectancy of a person with myelofibrosis depends on a number of factors, including the severity of the disease, the age of the patient and the response to treatment. In general, however, patients with myelofibrosis have a poor prognosis and a life expectancy of 5-10 years. There is no cure for myelofibrosis, but treatments are available to help relieve symptoms and improve quality of life. These include medication to reduce bone marrow scarring, blood transfusions to treat anaemia and pain relief. In some cases, a stem cell transplant may be recommended. If you have myelofibrosis, it's important to talk to your doctor about your treatment options and what you can do to manage your symptoms. There is no one-size-fits-all approach to treatment, and the best option for you will depend on your individual circumstances.

What does myeloproliferative mean?

A myeloproliferative neoplasm (MPN) is a type of cancer that affects the cells in the bone marrow that produce white blood cells. The three main types of MPNs are polycythemia vera, essential thrombocythemia, and primary myelofibrosis. MPNs can occur in people of any age, but are most common in adults over the age of 60. MPNs are caused by a genetic mutation that results in the overproduction of certain types of blood cells.

In polycythemia vera, for example, the body produces too many red blood cells. This can cause the blood to become thick and sticky, which can lead to problems such as blood clots. In essential thrombocythemia, the body produces too many platelets, which are the cells that help the blood to clot. This can increase the risk of bleeding. In primary myelofibrosis, the bone marrow produces too many white blood cells, which can cause the bone marrow to become crowded and unable to produce healthy blood cells. There are a number of symptoms that can be associated with MPNs, although not everyone will experience all of them. Common symptoms include fatigue, shortness of breath, dizziness, and headaches. More serious symptoms can include bleeding, bone pain, and organ damage. MPNs are usually diagnosed through a combination of physical examination, blood tests, and bone marrow biopsy. Treatment for MPNs can vary depending on the type and severity of the condition, but may include medication, blood transfusions, and, in some cases, bone marrow transplant.

Although leukaemia is a potentially fatal disease, there is reason to be hopeful. With advances in treatment and early detection, many people with leukaemia now enjoy long and healthy lives. With the support of loved ones and medical professionals, anyone diagnosed with leukaemia can face the challenges of the disease and emerge victorious.

What is the prognosis for myeloproliferative neoplasm?

A myeloproliferative neoplasm is a cancer of the blood and bone marrow. The prognosis for this type of cancer is often poor, as it is difficult to treat. Myeloproliferative neoplasms can be divided into four main types: myelodysplastic syndromes, myeloproliferative disorders, lymphomas, and Leukemias. Myelodysplastic syndromes are a group of blood disorders that affect the bone marrow. These disorders can cause the bone marrow to produce too few blood cells, or to produce blood cells that are abnormal. Myeloproliferative disorders are a group of blood disorders that cause the bone marrow to produce too many blood cells. Lymphomas are a type of cancer that affects the lymphocytes, which are a type of white blood cell. Leukemias are a type of cancer that affects the white blood cells. The prognosis for myeloproliferative neoplasms depends on the type of cancer, the stage of the cancer, and the age and health of the patient. Myelodysplastic syndromes and myeloproliferative disorders are often difficult to treat, and the prognosis is often poor. Lymphomas and Leukemias are often more responsive to treatment, but the prognosis is still often poor. The five-year survival rate for all types of myeloproliferative neoplasms is only about 20%. Patients with myeloproliferative neoplasms often require treatment with chemotherapy, radiation therapy, or both. Chemotherapy is the use of drugs to kill cancer cells. Radiation therapy is the use of high-energy beams to kill cancer cells. Both chemotherapy and radiation therapy can have side effects, such as nausea, vomiting, hair loss, and fatigue. Patients with myeloproliferative neoplasms often require a bone marrow transplant. A bone marrow transplant is a procedure in which healthy bone marrow cells are transplanted into the patient. The healthy cells can help the patient's bone marrow to produce normal blood cells. The success of a bone marrow transplant depends on many factors, such as the patient's age, the type of cancer, and the donor's age and health. Myeloproliferative neoplasms are difficult to treat and the prognosis is often poor. Treatment often requires chemotherapy, radiation therapy, or a bone marrow transplant. The five-year survival rate for all types of myeloproliferative neoplasms is only about 20%.

How long can you live with JAK2 mutation?

Although a person with a JAK2 mutation can live for many years, the disease can progress quickly and is often fatal. There is currently no cure for JAK2 mutation and no effective treatments available to slow down the progression of the disease. People with JAK2 mutations often experience symptoms such as fatigue, weight loss, easy bruising and bleeding, and bone pain. These symptoms can occur for many years before the disease progresses and becomes fatal. The average life expectancy for someone with a JAK2 mutation is between 5 and 10 years. However, some people with the disease have been known to live for 20 or more years. There are a few factors that can affect how long a person with a JAK2 mutation can live. These include the person's age, the severity of their symptoms, and their overall health. treatment options and how well they respond to treatment. Some people with JAK2 mutations are able to live relatively normal lives with the disease, while others can experience a rapid decline in their health.

What is the cause of myeloproliferative disorder?

Myeloproliferative neoplasms (MPN) are a group of cancers that affect the production of blood cells in the bone marrow. These disorders can cause an overproduction of one or more types of blood cells, which can lead to serious health problems. There are several possible causes of MPN, but the exact cause is unknown in most cases. However, there are some risk factors that have been linked to the development of these disorders. Some of the known risk factors for MPN include: • Having a family history of MPN or other blood disorders • Being exposed to certain chemicals or toxins, such as benzene • Having certain medical conditions, such as polycythemia vera (a disorder that causes the overproduction of blood cells) • Being diagnosed with a blood disorder at a young age • Being of certain ethnicities, such as Ashkenazi Jewish ancestry Although the exact cause of MPN is unknown, these disorders are thought to develop from abnormalities in the bone marrow. The bone marrow is the tissue in the center of bones that produces blood cells. Blood cells are produced through a process called hematopoiesis. In people with MPN, there is an abnormal change in the cells that line the bone marrow. This change causes the cells to grow and divide uncontrollably. The abnormal cells crowd out the healthy blood cells, which can lead to a number of problems. If you have MPN, you should see a doctor regularly to monitor your condition and to discuss treatment options. There is no cure for MPN, but treatment can help to manage the symptoms and prevent complications.

What are the first symptoms of myelofibrosis?

The first symptoms of myelofibrosis often include fatigue and weakness, as well as general flu-like symptoms such as fever, sweats, and chills. Many patients also experience bone pain, due to the overproduction of marrow. Enlargement of the spleen is another common symptom, as myelofibrosis can lead to excessive production of white blood cells. This can often cause a build-up of these cells in the spleen, leading to enlargement. In some cases, the spleen may become so enlarged that it presses on other organs, causing pain. Patients may also notice that they are bruise or bleed more easily than usual, as myelofibrosis can cause problems with blood clotting.

What is the end stage of myelofibrosis?

The end stage of myelofibrosis is characterized by the buildup of scar tissue in the bone marrow. This can cause problems with the production of blood cells, as well as lead to anemia and/or bleeding disorders. In some cases, the spleen may also become enlarged. Treatment options at this stage are limited, and may include bone marrow transplant or experimental therapies. There is no cure for myelofibrosis, and the disease often progresses to Leukemia.

How long can you have myelofibrosis without knowing?

Leukaemia is a cancer of the blood cells. The main types of blood cells are red blood cells, white blood cells, and platelets. Platelets help the blood to clot and white blood cells fight infection. Leukaemia can affect any of these blood cells, but the most common type is acute lymphoblastic leukaemia, which affects the white blood cells. Leukaemia is a cancer that starts in the bone marrow. The bone marrow is the spongy tissue inside the bones where blood cells are made. In leukaemia, the bone marrow produces too many abnormal blood cells. These abnormal cells crowd out the healthy blood cells, making it difficult for the blood to do its job. Leukaemia is usually a slowly progressing disease. For some people, the first sign of leukaemia is fatigue or easy bruising, which can be caused by a low number of platelets. Other people might have a fever, night sweats, or weight loss. These symptoms can be caused by a low number of white blood cells. If the leukaemia is more advanced, people might have shortness of breath, chest pain, or bone pain. Most people with leukaemia will need treatment with chemotherapy, radiation therapy, or a stem cell transplant. The type of treatment that is right for a person depends on the type of leukaemia they have, their age, and their overall health. Leukaemia can be a slow-progressing disease, which means that people can have it for a long time without knowing it. The first signs of leukaemia might be fatigue or easy bruising, which can be caused by a low number of platelets. Other people might have a fever, night sweats, or weight loss. These symptoms can be caused by a low number of white blood cells. If the leukaemia is more advanced, people might have shortness of breath, chest pain, or bone pain.

Can you live 20 years with myelofibrosis?

Myelofibrosis is a chronic blood disorder that can lead to bone marrow failure and a variety of other serious problems. There is currently no cure for myelofibrosis, and the average life expectancy for someone with the disease is five to ten years. However, some people with myelofibrosis have lived for 20 years or more. The key to living with myelofibrosis is to make sure that you are receiving the best possible treatment and to monitor your condition closely. There is currently no one standard treatment for myelofibrosis, so it is important to work with your doctor to find the treatment plan that is right for you. There are a variety of treatment options available, and new treatments are being developed all the time. In addition to treatment, there are a few things you can do to help manage your myelofibrosis and improve your quality of life. These include eating a healthy diet, getting regular exercise, and avoiding smoking. It is also important to stay connected with other people who have myelofibrosis. There are a number of support groups and online forums available, and connecting with others who are going through the same thing can be a great source of support. Myelofibrosis can be a difficult disease to live with, but it is possible to live a long and relatively healthy life with the condition. With the right treatment and support, you can manage your myelofibrosis and enjoy a good quality of life.

While leukaemia is a serious and often deadly disease, treatment has advanced significantly in recent years. Thanks to better understanding of the disease and improvements in technology, patients with leukaemia now have a much better chance of surviving and living a normal life.

* 9 7 8 1 7 7 6 9 6 9 5 6 2 *
SD - #0024 - 140926 - C0 - 229/152/17 - PB - 9781776969562 - Matt Lamination